D. ABECK W. BURGDORF H. CREMER (EDS.) **Common Skin Diseases in Children**

D. Abeck W. Burgdorf H. Cremer (Eds.)

Common Skin Diseases in Children

Diagnosis and Management

With 79 Colour Figures and 69 Tables

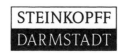

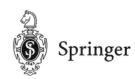

Univ. Prof. Dr. med. DIETRICH ABECK
Klinik und Poliklinik für Dermatologie
und Allergologie am Biederstein
Technische Universität München
Biedersteiner Str. 29, 80802 München
Germany

WALTER BURGDORF, MD
Traubinger Straße 45 A, 82327 Tutzing
Germany

Prof. Dr. med. HANSJOERG CREMER
ehm. Direktor der Städtischen Kinderklinik Heilbronn
Dittmarstr. 54, 74074 Heilbronn
Germany

ISBN 3-7985-1389-9 Steinkopff Verlag Darmstadt

Bibliographic information published by Die Deutsche Bibliothek
Die Deutsche Bibliothek lists this publication in the Deutsche Nationalbibliografie; detailed bibliographic data is available in the Internet at <http://dnb.ddb.de>.

Steinkopff Verlag Darmstadt
a member of BertelsmannSpringer Science+Business Media GmbH

http://www.steinkopff.springer.de

© Steinkopff Verlag Darmstadt 2003
Printed in Germany

Production Manager: K. Schwind
Cover designer: E. Kirchner
Typesetter: K+V Fotosatz GmbH, Beerfelden

SPIN 10912034   105/7231-5 4 3 2 1 0 – Printed on acid-free paper

Preface

Children with skin diseases may present to family physicians, pediatricians or dermatologists. In book we have tried to provide a concise and understandable source of information about common skin disorders which will be useful to any physician encountering children with cutaneous signs and symptoms.

We have concentrated on 26 common skin diseases which account for more than 90% of all skin-related doctor visits by children and adolescents, regardless of the orientation of the physician. The format of each chapter is uniform. The clinical description is accompanied by several typical photographs. The differential diagnostic approach with brief criteria is presented in a table. The major emphasis is on the treatment; we have tried to combine our long years of experience in pediatric dermatology with the international literature and especially more recent evidence-based studies. We have tried to present a range of therapeutic possibilities, but also give firm recommendations.

There have already been two successful German editions of this book. We hope that this first English edition also finds a receptive readership. We are committed to the concept that childhood skin diseases are best treated when all involved physicians have only one goal – the best possible care for all children. "Turf" battles between various specialties over aspects of care only harm our patients and in the end our own self-respect. The background of the three editors reflects this theme; there are two dermatologists, one German *(DA)* and one American *(WB)*, and a pediatrician *(HC)*. All of us have spent many years running special clinics in pediatric dermatology. The following younger colleagues have helped with the individual chapters –

Oliver Brandt	Matthias Moehrenschlager
Knut Brockow	Roland Remling
Heike Fesq	Tanja Schmidt
Ingeborg Forer	Christina Schnopp
Annette Heidelberger	Kerstin Strom
Bettina Heidtmann	Soehnke Thomsen
Martin Mempel	Lorenz B. Weigl

Although each is mentioned as an author of their individual chapters, we wish to acknowledge their help here as well. Each of them brought special knowledge and enthusiasm to this project.

We would also like to thank Steinkopff Verlag, Darmstadt, and especially Dr. Gertrud Volkert for their support of all stages of this project.

Most importantly, we hope that you the reader enjoy using this book and find it helpful in your daily practice. We will be gratified if on occasion this little book helps you reach a correct diagnosis or when the therapeutic guidance enables you to more effectively treat your young patients with disturbing skin diseases.

München, Tutzing and Heilbronn
Spring 2003

DIETRICH ABECK
WALTER BURGDORF
HANSJOERG CREMER

Contents

List of Contributors

Univ. Prof. Dr. med. Dietrich Abeck
Leitender Oberarzt
der Klinik und Poliklinik
für Dermatologie und Allergologie
am Biederstein
Technische Universität München
Biedersteiner Straße 29
80802 München, Germany

Oliver Brandt
Klinik und Poliklinik
für Dermatologie und Allergologie
am Biederstein
Technische Universität München
Biedersteiner Straße 29
80802 München, Germany

Dr. med. Knut Brockow
Klinik und Poliklinik
für Dermatologie und Allergologie
am Biederstein
Technische Universität München
Biedersteiner Straße 29
80802 München, Germany

Walter Burgdorf, MD
Traubinger Straße 45A
82327 Tutzing, Germany

Prof. Dr. med. Hansjoerg Cremer
ehm. Direktor der Städtischen
Kinderklinik Heilbronn
Dittmarstraße 54
74074 Heilbronn, Germany

Dr. med. Heike Fesq
Klinik und Poliklinik
für Dermatologie und Allergologie
am Biederstein
Technische Universität München
Biedersteiner Straße 29
80802 München, Germany

Dr. med. Ingeborg Forer
Klinik und Poliklinik
für Dermatologie und Allergologie
am Biederstein
Technische Universität München
Biedersteiner Straße 29
80802 München, Germany

Dr. med. Annette Heidelberger
Klinik und Poliklinik
für Dermatologie und Allergologie
am Biederstein
Technische Universität München
Biedersteiner Straße 29
80802 München, Germany

Dr. med. Bettina Heidtmann
Katholisches Kinderkrankenhaus
Wilhelmstift GmbH
Liliencronstraße 130
22149 Hamburg, Germany

Dr. med. Martin Mempel
Klinik und Poliklinik
für Dermatologie und Allergologie
am Biederstein
Technische Universität München
Biedersteiner Straße 29
80802 München, Germany

Dr. med. Matthias Moehrenschlager
Klinik und Poliklinik
für Dermatologie und Allergologie
am Biederstein
Technische Universität München
Biedersteiner Straße 29
80802 München, Germany

Dr. med. Roland Remling
Klinik und Poliklinik
für Dermatologie und Allergologie
am Biederstein
Technische Universität München
Biedersteiner Straße 29
80802 München, Germany

Dr. med. Tanja Schmidt
Klinik und Poliklinik
für Dermatologie und Allergologie
am Biederstein
Technische Universität München
Biedersteiner Straße 29
80802 München, Germany

Dr. med. Christina Schnopp
Klinik und Poliklinik
für Dermatologie und Allergologie
am Biederstein
Technische Universität München
Biedersteiner Straße 29
80802 München, Germany

Dr. med. Kerstin Strom
Läutwiesenweg 18
82205 Gilching, Germany

Dr. med. Soenke Thomsen
Harburger Ring 20
21073 Hamburg, Germany

Dr. med. Lorenz B. Weigl
Klinik und Poliklinik
für Dermatologie und Allergologie
am Biederstein
Technische Universität München
Biedersteiner Straße 29
80802 München, Germany

Chapter 1 Acne

K. Strom

Epidemiology

Acne is the most common skin disease during adolescence. Variants of acne also occur in infants and younger children. The incidence of neonatal acne (acne neonatorum) is estimated at 20%. Such patients have acne at birth or develop it in the first weeks of life. Most cases are mild and resolve spontaneously. The persistence of neonatal acne and the appearance of acne in childhood are both uncommon. Infantile acne (acne infantum) is an uncommon disease, but can be very severe (acne conglobata infantum) and may reflect an underlying endocrine disturbance, as well as be a marker for more severe acne during puberty. Almost every teenager develops at least a mild case of acne vulgaris. There are also exogenous types of acne or acneiform eruptions which can be seen in children such as acne cosmetica (also known as acne venenata) (from pomades or facial ointments), acne mechanica (from American football helmets and shoulder pads), steroid acne and chloracne.

Pathogenesis

Acne is a multifactorial disease. Genetics plays a role, as children of individuals with significant acne are more likely to have clinical problems. In addition, there are a variety of endogenous and exogenous factors which are important. There is an increased production of sebum coupled with a tendency to retain scales and lipids in the hair follicle. This facilitates colonization of the follicle and sebaceous glands by *Propionibacterium acnes*. These bacteria can have an inflammatory action by activating the complement cascade.

Hormonal factors such as rising androgen levels at the time of adrenarche have been shown to be responsible for acne in girls. In occasional cases of acne infantum, hormonal alterations in form of elevated levels of follicle stimulating hormone and testosterone can occasionally be found. In addition, some cases of the adrenogenital syndrome may present with acne.

Finally there are a number of possible topical triggers including corticosteroids, occlusive ointments and mechanical trauma. In rare cases, chloracne can be seen in children due to accidental contact with potent acnegenic dioxins like during the Soveto industrial accident in Italy.

Clinical Features

Acne only affects areas with sebaceous follicles; for this reason, in children the disease is generally limited to the face. Acne venenata infantum caused by occlusive ointments or pastes is an exception, as it can affect other body regions. Neonatal acne usually presents with closed comedones (white heads) and papulopustules (Fig. 1). Acne vulgaris typically has both closed comedones and open comedones (blackheads). These evolve into inflammatory papules and papulopustules. The usual patient shows all of the lesions in close proximity (Fig. 2). In acne conglobata, the most severe form of acne usually seen in teenage boys, additional

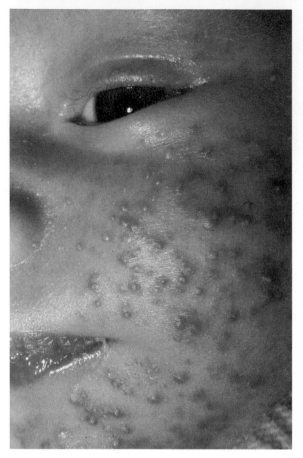

Fig. 1. Neonatal acne. Numerous papules as well as papulo-pustules on cheeks and chin.

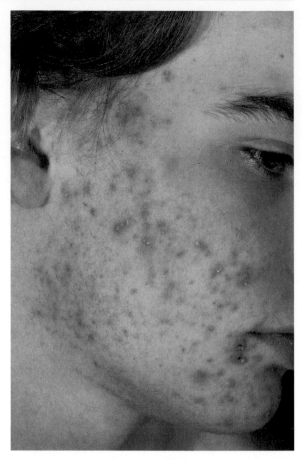

Fig. 2. Acne vulgaris. Open and closed comedones along with numerous papules and papulopustules.

findings include hemorrhagic crusted nodules and cysts. As the inflammatory lesions heal, they may leave pits, craters or keloids.

Symptoms

Usually acne is asymptomatic. Larger nodules or cystic lesions can itch or be painful.

Diagnosis

The diagnosis of acne is straightforward and already known to the patient. Special diagnostic procedures are not necessary. The history should include questions about possible exogenous factors.

A severe or therapy-resistant acne in childhood should suggest the possibility of

an underlying hormonal disturbance such as elevated androgen levels secondary to excessive ovarian or adrenal output of hormones. In such cases, free testosterone, dihydroepiandrosterone (DHEA), and dihydroepiandrosterone sulfate (DHEAS) should be determined. If any of these parameters are elevated, the dexamethasone suppression test is the test of choice to detect the source of the excess androgens.

Differential Diagnosis

The hallmark of acne is the presence of comedones, as well as a variety of inflammatory lesions. Table 1 shows the major differential diagnostic considerations. In infants, seborrheic dermatitis may appear similar but lacks comedones. In older children, peri-

Table 1. Differential diagnosis and important diagnostic clues for childhood acne

Diagnosis	Distinguishing Features
■ **Seborrheic dermatitis**	Shiny, greasy scales; no comedones
■ **Perioral dermatitis**	Perioral, periocular and perinasal localization (with zone of sparing), no comedones; often caused by topical corticosteroids
■ **Rosacea**	Papules, pustules, telangiectases and persistent erythema on the cheeks, nose, and chin; no comedones; occasionally caused by topical corticosteroids

Table 2. General therapeutic approach for the various forms of acne in children

■ **Neonatal acne**	No treatment usually needed; perhaps azelaic acid cream
■ **Infantile acne**	Combined use of topical antibiotics/ antiseptics and retinoids; systemic isotretinoin only for acne conglobata infantum
■ **Acne vulgaris**	Combined use of topical antibiotics/ antiseptics; systemic minocycline if not responsive; systemic isotretinoin for severe cases
■ **Acne cosmetica**	Discontinue the triggering agent(s); topical retinoids
■ **Steroid acne**	Discontinue topical corticosteroids; attempt to reduce dose of systemic corticosteroids (the usual trigger); topical retinoids or metronidazole usually most effective

oral dermatitis poses the same challenge but once again lacks comedones and has a slightly different localization.

Therapy

The localization and severity of the acne determine whether topical therapy alone suffices or whether systemic measures should also be undertaken. Facial comedones and papulopustules can usually be treated topically. Nodular and cystic lesions, especially on the trunk, usually require additional systemic measures. The rare children with acne conglobata infantum require systemic treatment. In contrast, neonatal acne is usually self-limited, requiring either no treatment or mild measures (Table 2).

One should never underestimate the emotional impact of acne on young patients. Often they need a friend with an encouraging word almost as much as a prescription. There may be marked discrepancies between the observed degree of involvement and the patient's own assessment of their disease, its severity and its effect on their life.

■ Topical Therapy

The topical treatment of acne is directed against the follicular occlusion, the microbial agents and the excessive sebum.

■ **Cleansing Products.** Sebum production cannot be influenced by topical measures. Frequent cleansing of the skin with synthetic detergents (syndets) or soaps, as well as wiping with alcoholic solutions, serve to remove the surface lipids. Syndets are generally less irritating and widely used in Europe. Some prefer to use an antiseptic alcoholic solution (such as 1% chlorhexidine gluconate in 40% isopropyl alcohol) following washing. Patients should be counseled against too frequent or too aggressive washing, especially using abrasive soaps or similar products. The irritation makes the subsequent therapy more difficult.

■ **Antibiotics.** Topical antibiotics reduce the levels of *Propionibacterium acnes* and also have an anti-inflammatory action. They should not be used as a monotherapy in order to reduce the risk of the development of resistant stains of *Propionibacterium acnes* and other resident flora such as coagulase-negative staphylococci. In addition, the combined use of topical antibiotics and antiseptics is clinically more effective than either approach alone.

The most widely employed topical antibiotics are erythromycin, clindamycin and tetracycline.

Topical tetracycline discolors the skin and causes fluorescence under black lights, such as might be found in a disco. In contrast, topical clindamycin and erythromycin have few if any side effects and are comparable in effect. Both are available in a variety of forms including alcoholic solutions and gels. Erythromycin is also available combined with either benzoyl peroxide or zinc.

In Europe, erythromycin is often compounded. Possible formulations include:

■ Alcohol-based 2% erythromycin gel (NRF 11.84.)
Rx_
Erythromycin	2.0 g
Anhydrous citric acid	0.155 g
Ethanol 96% (V/V)	45.0 g
Hydroxypropylcellulose 400	5.0 g
Distilled water ad	100.0 mL

■ Alcohol-based 2% erythromycin solution (NRF 11.78.)
Rx_
Erythromycin	2.0 g
Anhydrous citric acid	0.155 g
Ethanol 96% (V/V)	45.0 g
Distilled water ad	100.0 mL

■ **Antiseptics.** The two major antiseptic agents, benzoyl peroxide and azelaic acid, have both an antimicrobial and comedolytic action. Benzoyl peroxide is available in 2.5, 5.0 and 10.0% concentrations, as a water-based or alcoholic gel, cream, lotion, or liquid soap. We favor the 2.5% concentration for children, as the 5–10% products cause more irritation and are only slightly more effective. In teenagers with oily skin, the higher concentrations in a more drying vehicle such as a alcoholic gel may be most appropriate. If marked irritation occurs, it may well be that the patient is using too much of the product or using it too often. Allergic contact dermatitis to benzoyl peroxide is quite uncommon.

Azelaic acid has a wide variety of actions, as it is not only antiseptic but also inhibits the conversion of testosterone to $5\text{-}a$-dihydrotestosterone. Although the literature suggests that azelaic acid is comparable in effectiveness to benzoyl peroxide, we have found it to be somewhat less helpful. We employ it most often in children with mild acne and easily irritated skin.

■ **Keratolytic Agents.** The topical retinoids (vitamin A acid derivatives) are the mainstay of keratolytic or comedolytic therapy. They normalize the follicular keratinization process and disrupt microcomedones before they can evolve into clinical lesions. For this reason, topical retinoids are of benefit in all stages of acne. The classic topical retinoid is tretinoin, which is available in concentrations of 0.025, 0.05 and 0.1% provided as creams, gels and solutions. All the products tend to be irritating, cause dryness, erythema and scaling. One must be cautious about concentrations because a 0.05% gel is usually more irritating than a 0.1% cream. In addition, two products from different manufacturers with the same concentration of tretinoin may vary widely in their irritating effects. Solutions are the most irritating and not often used in children.

In addition to counseling the patient and their parents about irritation, one must warn them that their acne may worsen for the first 4–6 weeks as the comedones are attacked by the product. It is wise to only use topical retinoids once daily in the evening, because of the risk of photosensitization. Enough of the product remains on the skin, even following washing the next morning, that the patients should be careful and use a sunscreen. Some patients only tolerate an every other day application.

Two newer retinoids are available – adapalene and isotretinoin. Both are similar in properties, less irritating than tretinoin without phototoxicity, but in our hands also somewhat less effective. Both are useful in children with mild comedonal acne who do not tolerate tretinoin.

■ Systemic Therapy

■ **Antibiotics.** Systemic antibiotics are not superior to topical application and therefore topical antibiotic treatment should be considered first. Systemic antibiotics both reduce levels of *Propionibacterium acnes* and also have an anti-inflammatory effect by inhibiting neutrophil chemotaxis. They first achieve their maximal effects after 6–8 weeks of treatment. Treatment with oral antibiotics should always be combined with topical measures.

Minocycline is the antibiotic of choice for treating acne. A daily dosage of 100 mg is recommended given for a period of three months (maximum six months). The drug is very lipophilic leading to nearly complete intestinal absorption. Because of reports of minocycline-related hepatitis, serum sickness and lupus erythematosus, the CBC and baseline liver function tests should be monitored prior to starting therapy and at monthly or bimonthly intervals.

Minocycline and other tetracyclines should not be used in children less than 9 years of age because they can cause irreversible discoloration of teeth, damage to dental enamel and reversible inhibition of bone growth. Alternative systemic antibiotics include erythromycin and clindamycin. Because erythromycin is often associated with development of resistance by *Propionibacterium acnes*, it should always be combined with a topical antiseptic or keratolytic agent. The usual dosage is 30–50 mg/kg in 2–4 divided doses. We only employ clindamycin on rare occasions because of the small but definite risk of pseudomembranous colitis.

■ **Isotretinoin.** The vitamin A acid analog, isotretinoin or 13-cis retinoic acid, is dramatically effective in acne. It is comedolytic, reduces sebum levels (secondarily reducing levels of *Propionibacterium acnes*) and has an anti-inflammatory action. Isotretinoin has one major side effect which has limited its use and caused an array of regulatory problems. It is a potent teratogen, so that it can only be used by girls and women who are practicing strict contraception. Often this is a difficult goal to achieve in teenagers, as they may not be entirely truthful about their sexual practices, especially if their parents are involved in the discussion. Other side effects relevant in children include dry skin and mucosal surfaces (eyes, nasal mucosa), growth retardation and the DISH syndrome (disseminated idiopathic skeletal hyperostoses). In adults, elevated triglyceride levels and altered liver function may also be significant clinical factors. We only employed systemic isotretinoin for severe acne in teenagers, as well as on occasion for the rare acne conglobata infantum. The usual dosage is 0.3–0.7 mg/kg for 4–6 months, trying to reach a total dose of 120 mg/kg, the level at which recurrences become less likely.

References

Berson D. S., Shalita A. R.: The treatment of acne: the role of combination therapies. Journal of the American Academy of Dermatology 32:S31–S41 (1995)

Goulden V., Layton A. M., Cuncliffe W. J.: Long-term safety of isotretinoin as a treatment for acne vulgaris. British Journal of Dermatology 131:360–363 (1994)

Jansen T., Burgdorf W. H., Plewig G.: Pathogenesis and treatment of acne in childhood. Pediatric Dermatology 14:17–21 (1997)

Lehmann H. P., Robinson K. A., Andrews J. S., Holloway V., Goodman S.: Acne therapy: a methodologic review. J Am Acad Dermatol 47:231–240 (2002)

Lehucher-Ceyrac D., Weber-Buisset M. J.: Isotretinoin and acne in practice: a prospective analysis of 188 cases over 9 years. Dermatology 186:123–128 (1993)

Lucky A. W.: Acne therapy in infancy and childhood. Dermatologic Therapy 6:74–81 (1998)

Plewig G., Albrecht G., Henz B. M., Meigel W., Schöpf E., Stadler R.: Systemische Behandlung der Akne mit Isotretinoin: Aktueller Stand. Hautarzt 48:881–885 (1997)

Rothmann K. F.: Acne update. Dermatologic Therapy 2:98–110 (1997)

Somech R., Arav-Boger R., Assia A., Spirer Z., Jurgenson U.: Complications of minocycline therapy for acne vulgaris: case reports and review of the literature. Ped Dermatol 16:469–472 (1999)

CHAPTER 2 Alopecia Areata

M. MÖHRENSCHLAGER, L. B. WEIGL

Epidemiology

The incidence of alopecia areata is about 17/ 100,000. Most patients are children and young adults; both sexes are affected equally. Occasional familial cases have been described. There is an association with atopic dermatitis, vitiligo, and thyroid disease.

Pathogenesis

The cause of alopecia areata remains a mystery. A variety of possibilities have been suggested including autoimmune phenomena, endocrine and neurological disturbances, vascular changes and psychological factors.

Clinical Features

Usually alopecia areata has a dramatic and easily diagnosed clinical appearance. Typically there are one or more sharply bordered, round or oval areas with complete hair loss and prominent follicular openings (Fig. 3). The usual location is the occipital or parietal scalp. The individual patches may coalesce. A classic clinical sign is the presence of exclamation point hairs, which can be found at the periphery of the ivory patches which may also show slight inflammatory erythema. These hairs are broken off distally, have a narrowed shaft and then sometimes a thickened region directly at the scalp level, thus, fancifully resembling the printer's symbol of !.

In the ophiasis variant of alopecia areata, accounting for less than 5% of cases, the hair loss occurs in the area covered by the band of a hat, usually starting in the occipital region but extending temporally. Alopecia areata totalis refers to the complete loss of the scalp hairs and occurs in 5–10% of cases. In contrast, patients with the much more rare (1% of cases) alopecia areata universalis suffer the loss of other body hairs, such as eyelashes, eyebrows, axillary and pubic hairs.

Another associated sign is the presence of pitted nails which can be found in up to 60% of cases, depending on how carefully one searches. The nail changes can appear long before the hair loss. In other instances, children have pitted nails and never develop alopecia areata. These changes are designated trachyonychia. Nail involvement, especially if prominent, is more likely to be associated with severe alopecia areata.

Poor prognostic signs include onset during early childhood, widespread or complete hair loss, nail involvement and atopic dermatitis.

Symptoms

While the scalp lesions are asymptomatic, the psychological trauma is often severe and may be the most dramatic problem on presentation.

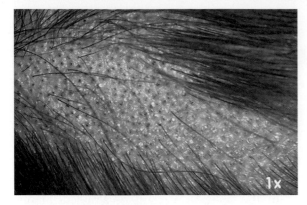

Fig. 3. Alopecia areata. Oval area of complete hair loss with retained follicular orifices.

Diagnosis

The diagnosis can usually be made with the history and clinical examination. The exclamation point hairs are an especially helpful sign. A trichogram (forceful epilation and microscopic analysis of 25–50 hairs to determine their growth status) is not clinically necessary and often traumatizes the young patient. A scalp biopsy and histologic examination may be useful in cases which are clinically unclear, as when trichotillomania or scarring alopecia (as with lupus erythematosus or lichen planus) is suspected.

Differential Diagnosis

The major differential diagnostic considerations are shown in Table 3. The most common challenge is identifying trichotillomania; the major differences are that here the lesions are less regular, the hair loss is not as complete, and the remaining hairs have variable lengths (Fig. 4).

Therapy

The various therapeutic options are summarized in Table 4.

Table 3. Differential diagnosis of alopecia areata

Diagnosis	Distinguishing Features
■ **Aplasia cutis**	Solitary or multiple areas with complete absence of hair, present at birth, with no tendency to change or spread
■ **Alopecia triangularis**	Congenital absence of hairs bilaterally in the fronto-temporal area, with no tendency to change or spread
■ **Tinea capitis**	Erythematous, scaly patches with positive KOH examination and fungal culture
■ **Trichotillomania**	Irregularly bordered, usually solitary, areas with hair loss and remaining hairs of varying lengths; occasional follicular hemorrhages; often occurs contralateral to the dominant hand
■ **Traction alopecia**	Thinning and loss of hairs in a symmetrical way along the forehead, temples or occipital region because of tension caused by hair style (pony tail, tight braided styles in blacks)
■ **Infantile alopecia**	Patch of hair loss on the occiput in young infants who spread a great deal of time lying on their back; a form of traumatic alopecia

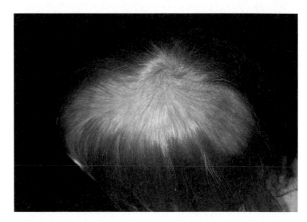

Fig. 4. Trichotillomania. Thinning of the scalp hairs which have varying lengths. The follicular orifices are still present.

■ **Watchful Waiting.** Each and every therapy for alopecia areata must be evaluated bearing in mind that about 60% of patients with a single new lesion will experience complete regrowth within one year without any treatment. Thus, if the parents are in agreement, watchful waiting is often a useful option if the child is not greatly disturbed by the hair loss.

Table 4. Treatment of alopecia areata in childhood

Treatment	Procedure
■ **Watchful waiting**	No therapy, as most cases in children resolve spontaneously
■ **Topical corticosteroids**	Medium to high potency topical corticosteroid creams or solutions are applied to the lesion nightly for 3 weeks, followed by a 1 week therapy pause. At least 3–4 cycles are needed
■ **Systemic corticosteroids**	0.5–1.0 mg/kg methyl prednisolone daily for 14 days, followed by alternate day administration with gradual tapering. Many side effects and frequent recurrences
■ **Short contact anthralin**	0.5% anthralin cream is applied for 5 minutes and then removed by shampooing. The exposure is increased by 5 minutes every three days until 45–60 minutes is reached. Then the concentration is increased to 0.75%, 1%, 1.25%, 1.5% and 2% with the same pattern of prolonging the time
■ **Overnight anthralin**	Treatment started with 1/64% anthralin ointment which is applied nightly and removed in the morning. After two week intervals, dosage increased to 1/32%, 1/16%, 1/8%, 1/4%, 1/2%, 3/4% and 1%
■ **Diphenyl-cyclopropenone (DCP)**	Starting 14 days after initial sensitization with 2% DCP, a far more dilute solution (usually 0.00001% DCP) is applied once weekly, with the goal of maintaining a mild contact dermatitis for 3 days. If no reaction occurs, the concentration can be increased. Treatment is usually required for at least one year

Alopecia Areata

■ **Topical Corticosteroids.** If treatment is desired, topical corticosteroids are the method of choice for limited disease. Mid to high potency agents in cream or solution form are best. The product is applied once daily to the bald area and 1 cm into the surrounding hair, usually in the evening. If a solution proves drying, one can switch to a cream. When larger areas are involved, occlusion with a disposable shower cap may be helpful. We treat nightly for three weeks, followed by a one week pause. Occasionally one sees a corticosteroid-induced folliculitis; otherwise side effects are not a problem. A number of cycles, at least 3–4, are required.

The intralesional injection of corticosteroids is painful and we rarely employ this method. Children older than 10 years of age can usually tolerate it, if EMLA cream is applied one hour before the planned injection to minimize the pain of the procedure. We attempt to inject 0.1 mL of triamcinolone acetonide (2.5–5.0 mg/mL) in a strictly intradermal location at 1–2 cm intervals through the lesion especially at the periphery. Another possibility is to raise several wheals, each with 0.3–0.4 mL, and then massage the fluid into the tissue. The maximum amount to be injected is 2 mL. The injections should be repeated every 4–6 weeks.

■ **Anthralin.** Irritant contact dermatitis can be induced with the application of anthralin, an standard psoriasis medication. Today it appears that in addition to its irritant effects, anthralin may also have an immunomodulatory role, blocking Langerhans cell function.

We prefer anthralin therapy for children with more widespread disease. It has been safely employed for this problem for over 100 years. The treatment regimen is complex and requires cooperative patients and parents, because if anthralin is misused, it causes a severe irritant dermatitis. Anthralin therapy is time consuming and requires multiple visits to the physician, but can be carried out at home, in contrast to treatment with diphenylcyclopropenone.

We prefer short contact anthralin therapy, starting with a 0.5% preparation which must be compounded by the pharmacist in an ointment or emollient cream base. It is applied for 5 minutes daily and then removed by shampooing. The exposure time is increased by 5 minutes every three days until an exposure time of 45–60 minutes is reached. At this point, the concentration is increased to 0.75%, 1%, 1.25%, 1.5% and 2.0%, each time following the same protocol for increasing the time of exposure starting at 5 minutes.

If the overnight regimen is selected, much lower concentrations must be employed. We usually start with a 1/64% preparation and increase the strength every two weeks, following the increments 1/32%, 1/16%, 1/8%, 1/4%, 1/2%, 3/4% and 1%. Anthralin discolors bedding and clothing so the patient should wear a shower cap overnight. Anthralin also discolors the skin, so whoever applies the product should wear disposable plastic gloves. The discoloration resolves, once therapy is discontinued. If the anthralin causes too much irritation, therapy can be interrupted for a few days and a topical corticosteroid cream employed, perhaps with moist compresses. Once the irritation is resolved, the patient can re-start the anthralin at the last level which was tolerated without problems and then slowly advance again.

■ **Diphenylcyclopropenone.** In recent years, topical immunotherapy has become well-established for alopecia areata. We generally use 2,3-diphenylcyclopropenone (DCP), although other agents (dinitrochlorobenzole, squaric acid dibutylester) are available. While DCP is not officially approved for treating alopecia areata, it appears safe, as it is non-mutagenic in the Ames test and shows no signs of teratogenicity or organ toxicity in animal testing. Nonetheless, because of its immunomodulatory role, we reserve its use to older children (>12 years of age) with at least 30% hair loss in whom other modalities have failed. In most instances DCP therapy is carried in academic centers with considerable experience in treating alopecia areata.

The child is initially sensitized to DCP by applying a 2% solution to a 4×4 cm patch of normal skin. Two weeks later we start applying a 0.00001% solution of DCP to the involved area weekly. We try to induce a mild allergic contact dermatitis in the area of alopecia areata with erythema and pruritus for 2–3 days. If there is no reaction, one can gradually increase the concentration, first to 0.0001%, and then over months up to a maximum of 2% (almost never needed). The patient and the physician or nurse who applies the DCP must be sure to avoid contact with the solution, or they may get an allergic contact dermatitis. The hair should not be shampooed for 48 hours. The usual duration of treatment is at least one year.

Just as with anthralin, a clinically significant contact dermatitis may develop, requiring discontinuing DCP and application of topical corticosteroids. When the reaction has resolved, one can start DCP again at an accordingly lower concentration. Some patients receiving DCP have so much pruritus that they have difficulty sleeping; usually a sedating H1 antihistamine is sufficient to manage the problem. Nuchal and retroauricular lymphadenopathy may also be seen, but it is reversible and not an indication to stop treatment.

■ **Systemic Corticosteroids.** Systemic corticosteroids are occasionally appropriate for very severe alopecia areata or in patients who have failed to respond to other approaches. We give 0.5–1.0 mg/kg of methyl prednisolone daily for 14 days, and then switch to alternate day therapy and taper the level of the corticosteroids over 4–6 weeks. The Olson-Carney-Turney protocol suggests 0.75 mg/kg of methyl prednisolone daily for one week, then reducing the dose by 1/8th each week for four weeks, and finally administering 1/8th of the original dose every 3rd day for 14 days. Both regimens have numerous side effects, including hypertension, pseudotumor cerebri, purpura, growth retardation, striae, telangiectases, acne, hirsutism and telogen effluvium. In addition, in over 50% of the cases with a satisfactory regrowth, hair loss reoccurs once the corticosteroids are stopped. For these reasons, it is difficult to be enthusiastic about systemic corticosteroids for alopecia areata.

■ **Topical Photochemotherapy.** While some groups endorse topical PUVA (application of 8-methoxy psoralen solution followed by increasing amounts of UVA irradiation), we have found this approach ineffective and do not employ it.

■ **Minoxidil.** Topical minoxidil is available in a 2% solution for the treatment of male pattern baldness. The commercial product, and other solutions containing up to 5% minoxidil, have been endorsed for alopecia areata. In most studies, the medication is applied b.i.d.; while some hair growth is often seen, cosmetically acceptable results are uncommon. Since minoxidil is not approved for this indication in Germany, we recommend it be used for alopecia areata only in appropriately controlled clinical studies.

■ **Future Prospects.** Several immunomodulators (systemic cyclosporine A, topical tacrolimus and pimecrolimus) as well as cytokines (interferon-α) have been tried in alopecia areata. Until results of clinical studies are available, we cannot recommend their use in children.

■ **Supportive Measures.** There are many ways to hide a lesion of alopecia areata while waiting for spontaneous improvement or effective therapeutic results. Creative hair styling, wearing head bands or even currently stylish baseball caps should all be considered. In children with alopecia areata totalis and universalis, where regrowth is unlikely, the physician should work with the health insurance company to obtain a high quality wig for the patient. The devastating emotional effects of clinically obvious or severe alopecia areata should never be forgotten. These unfortunate children need as much additional support as the physician and his staff can possibly provide.

References

Happle R.: Topical immunotherapy in alopecia areata. Journal of Investigative Dermatology 96:71S–72S (1991)

Hull S.M., Pepall L., Cuncliffe W.J.: Alopecia areata in children: response to treatment with diphencyprone. British Journal of Dermatology 125:164–168 (1991)

Madani S., Shapiro J.: Alopecia areata update. Journal of the American Academy of Dermatology 42:549–566 (2000)

Niedner R.: Glukokortikoide in der Dermatologie. Deutsches Ärzteblatt 93:A-2863–2872 (1996)

Olsen E.A., Carson S.C., Turney E.A.: Systemic steroids with or without 2% minoxidil in the treatment of alopecia areata. Archives of Dermatology 128:1467–1473 (1992)

Papadopoulos A.J., Schwartz R.A., Janniger C.K.: Alopecia areata. Pathogenesis, diagnosis, and therapy. Am J Clin Dermatol 1:101–105 (2000)

Price V.H.: Treatment of hair loss. The New England Journal of Medicine 341:964–973 (1999)

Sahn E.E.: Alopecia areata in childhood. Seminars in Dermatology 14:9–14 (1995)

Schroeder T.L., Levy M.L.: Treatment of hair loss disorders in children. Dermatological Therapy 2:84–92 (1997)

Schuttelaar M.L., Hamstra J.J., Plinck E.P., Peereboom-Wynia J.D.R., Vuzevski V.D., Mulder P.G.H., Oranje A.P.: Alopecia areata in children: treatment with diphencyprone. British Journal of Dermatology 135:581–585 (1996)

Schwartz R.A., Janniger C.K.: Alopecia areata. Pediatric Dermatology 59:238–241 (1997)

Thiers B.H.: Alopecia areata. Clinical Dermatology 2:1–15 (1989)

CHAPTER 3 Arthropod Bite and Sting Reactions

R. REMLING

Epidemiology

Reactions to arthropod bites and stings are a common problem as arthropods are widely distributed and many have life cycles which require them to feed from other animals, including humans. Others have biting or stinging devices which they use for defense. Many more noxious arthropods are found in warmer climates. We will concentrate only on those organisms found in temperate western Europe; most of these animals are also found in the continental USA. Although every individual is at risk, those living in close living conditions, lacking simple protective measures (screens, for example) and practicing poor hygiene are at greatest risk.

Pathogenesis

■ **Immunologic Reactions.** The following reactions following an arthropod assault are immunologically mediated:

- IgE-mediated Type I reaction with urticaria and possible anaphylaxis.
- IgG-mediated Type III reaction with localized or generalized vasculitis.
- Type IV reaction mediated by sensitized T cells leading to dermatitis.

The typical course of local allergic reactions is that the initial assault results in a delayed reaction after 24–48 hours. Subsequent exposures lead to an acute often urticarial reaction with later dermatitic changes. In the case of repeated assaults, such as a bee-keeper, a degree of immunologic tolerance may develop.

A special type of immunologic reaction is the pseudolymphoma, in which case a firm persistent red-brown nodule develops at a bite or sting site. Typical triggers are tick bites, scabies and flea bites. Microscopic examination reveals a dense reactive lymphocytic infiltrate which may persist for many months.

■ **Non-immunologic Reactions**

- Reactions caused by pharmacologically active toxins contained in the arthropod's saliva or "administered" by special delivery systems, leading to both local and systemic affects. The latter are more likely with scorpion and certain spider stings
- Mechanical trauma following damaging the skin during a blood meal (horse flies, ticks) or as part of protective response (spiders, scorpions)
- Skin invasion by *Sarcoptes scabiei*
- Secondary infection of the wound either by bacteria transmitted by the arthropod (wasps, flies) or because of scratching by the victim
- Transmission of infectious diseases (ticks → borreliosis, meningoencephalitis; mosquitoes → variety of viral infections).

Clinical Features

The cutaneous reactions to bites and stings depend on the arthropod, the site of the bite, the degree of sensitization and the victim's immune status. The correct diagnosis requires correlation of the clinical picture with the history to suggest the most likely assailant. The three most common problems are discussed in separate chapters: lice in Chapter 10, ticks in Chapter 12 and scabies in Chapter 19.

■ **Bedbugs.** *Cimex lectularius*, the common bedbug, is a 3–5 mm true bug, which is active at night and requires only one blood meal weekly. It usually lives in crevices in the floor, in upholstery or in picture frames. Occasionally one hears of someone acquiring not only a nice antique but also bedbugs from a "flea market." The bedbugs tend to drop from the ceiling onto their victim. Their classic clinical trademark is a series of linearly arranged urticarial pruritic papules (Fig. 5) which are acquired during the night and found on exposed skin. When examined with diascopy (pressing a glass slide or spatula on the skin), they often reveal a central hemorrhagic punctum. Examining the bedding and bed clothes maybe helpful, as spots of blood can be seen.

■ **Fleas.** The host specificity of fleas is minimal, so human fleas can attack animals and vice versa. The human flea, *Pulex irritans,* is one of the great athletes of the animal world. Although it is only 5–7 mm long, it can jump up to 50 cm high and 60 cm in distance. It feeds several times a day and can ingest its blood meal with amazing rapidity. These fleas avoid light at all costs, hiding in crevices during the day, and spring onto the victims at night. They tend to feed on covered sites.

Flea bites are urticarial lesions which usually have a bit of blue-red hemorrhage (purpura pulicosa). They are usually irregularly distributed on the body. In children, they may sometimes be papulo-vesicular and difficult to distinguish from strophulus.

■ **Hymenoptera.** Members of this order have two pairs of membranous wings connected by a small hook. Included in the group are

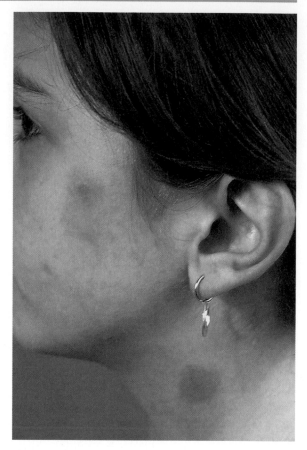

Fig. 5. Bedbug bites. Nummular erythematous papules with central vesicle along almost linear pattern from cheek to neck.

bees, bumble bees, wasps and hornets. They sting with a barbed apparatus on their posterior section which is attached to a sac containing toxin.

Bee stings are frequently seen on the feet of children who have walked through a meadow or lawn. One should examine a bee sting carefully, as the stinger may still be in place. If so, it should be removed carefully with a small tweezers, carefully avoiding manipulating the attached toxin sack. Wasps tend more often to bite on the head, neck and arms, as they are attracted to outdoor food and drink and, thus, come into conflict with humans. Occasionally a wasp may land in a glass and then be ingested when the contents are drunk.

The local reaction to stings is well known to all – pain, erythema, swelling and in

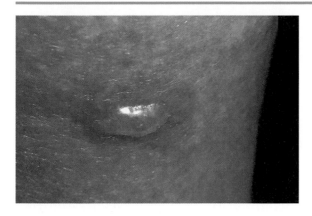

Fig. 6. Bullous mosquito bite reaction. Tense clear blister on erythematous base.

some cases blister formation. Such a chain of events in the mouth can lead to obstruction. In addition, systemic reactions can occur within just a few minutes leading to pruritus, diffuse urticaria, anaphylaxis and even circulatory collapse in allergic people.

■ **Diptera.** Included in this large order are flies and mosquitoes. They are characterized by having just one pair of membranous wings and a pair of club-shaped balancing organs known as halteres. Mosquitoes are most active in the early morning and early evening; they bite exposed areas. They are most common when small amounts of standing water are available, as these are their preferred breeding sites.

The initial mosquito bite is an pruritic erythematous wheal which evolves into a firm papule persisting for hours to days. On occasion, the bite may become bullous (Fig. 6) or lead to a more severe local reaction with erythema, warmth and swelling, usually on a limb. Secondary impetiginization is common as a result of scratching.

■ **Trombidiosis.** The harvest mite (Trombicula) larvae appear in great numbers in the warm summer months. They are found on flowers, shrubs, vines and trees, dropping off to land on their victims. They then move until they encounter resistance from a collar, elastic band or belt, at which time they take a blood meal. The typical clinical findings

are a series of grouped intensely pruritic wheals without hemorrhage arranged along such a barrier line. Often there is a delay of several hours before signs and symptoms begin, so that the patient or parent does not associate the lesions with the outdoors. The lesions develop into firm erythematous nodules which persist for weeks and are not influenced by therapy.

■ **Cheyletiella.** These animal mites, also known as walking mange, are transferred from cats, dogs and horses, as well as some wild mammals. There is usually a latent period, followed by the development of pruritic, disseminated papules or papulo-vesicles, most commonly on areas which have been in contact with animals (arms, trunk). The history of animal contact coupled with an examination of the suspect animal which usually has readily visible moving "scale" make the diagnosis. These mites do not burrow into human skin, but leave after biting.

■ **Bird mites.** Chicken and bird mites (*Dermanyssus gallinae seu avium*) reside in the nests of the hosts and then feed at night when the birds are nesting. They are typically transferred to humans who clean chicken coops or bird nests, such as pigeon breeders. Clinically the bites are small pruritic papulo-vesicular lesions on the hands and arms. With repeated exposure, both dermatitic skin changes and an allergic asthma can develop. The history of occupational or avocational exposure is the best clue.

Diagnosis

The diagnosis of arthropod bites and stings is not as easy as it sounds in the text. Patients seem more annoyed by this diagnosis than almost any other; often they express the attitude, "If it were just bites or stings, I would have known it and not come to the doctor". In addition, the physician must often say that they suspect a bite, rather than being definite.

Differential Diagnosis

The main symptom of all arthropod assaults is pruritus. The main differential diagnostic considerations include urticaria and strophulus. Occasionally erythema multiforme can be mistaken for multiple insect bites. But usually there is a history of herpes simplex, other infectious disease or intake of some medication. Strophulus (also known as prurigo simplex acuta) is an difficult concept; sometimes following an arthropod assault, the patient, almost always a child, develops numerous papulo-vesicles which are pruritic and later form crusts. The key is that the lesions are reactive, as not all develop at sites of assault. It can be very difficult to separate strophulus from multiple bites. Other possibilities include viral exanthems and drug eruptions, both of which can occasionally be papulo-vesicular. Longstanding dermatitic bite reactions can resemble contact dermatitis or even prurigo-like lesions in atopic dermatitis. The most important task is to try and make an educated guess as to what type of arthropod could be responsible, in order to facilitate further management (Table 5).

Table 5. Differential diagnosis of the most common arthropod bites and stings

Causative Agent	Distinguishing Features	Differential Diagnosis
■ **Head lice**	Presence of lice or nits, especially on occiput; dermatitis of the nape	Atopic dermatitis, contact dermatitis, tinea capitis, psoriasis
■ **Bedbugs**	Social history; linear urticarial lesions with hemorrhagic punctae on exposed areas	Urticaria, strophulus, urticarial drug eruption, other arthropod reactions
■ **Fleas**	Asymmetrical pattern of bites on covered skin; papulo-vesicles; urticarial lesions with central hemorrhage	Urticaria, strophulus, varicella
■ **Hymenoptera (bees, wasps, hornets)**	History; edematous painful erythema with possible blisters; generalized urticaria and anaphylaxis possible	Urticaria, erysipelas, toxic dermatitis; other types of anaphylaxis
■ **Diptera (mosquitoes, flies)**	History; urticarial erythematous papules on exposed areas; usually no hemorrhage; scratching with crusts and secondary impetiginization	Urticaria, strophulus, impetigo, other arthropod reactions
■ **Scabies**	Family history; intense pruritus worse at night; erythematous papules and tunnels; typically interdigital, genital, flexural, perimamillary; mite can be identified	Atopic dermatitis, seborrheic dermatitis, contact dermatitis; with palms and soles involved, infantile acropustulosis, dyshidrotic dermatitis
■ **Trombidiosis**	Occurs in summer; outdoor exposure; urticarial papules and sero-papules along clothing lines and body folds; no hemorrhage or tunnels	Urticaria, strophulus
■ **Cheyletiella**	History of animal exposure; disseminated pruritic papules on arms and trunk; often delay following pet contact; no tunnels	Strophulus, drug reaction
■ **Chicken, bird mites**	History of bird exposure; urticarial and papulo-vesicular lesions on exposed areas; no tunnels	Urticaria, drug reaction, contact dermatitis
■ **Ticks**	History of outdoor exposure; presence of tick	Other arthropod reactions; other pseudolymphomas

Table 6. Treatment of arthropod bites and stings

Clinical Features	Treatment
■ **One or few lesions**	Topical corticosteroids or local anesthetics (5% polidocanol in cream base)
■ **Disseminated lesions**	As above plus systemic antihistamine
■ **Generalized lesions and/or systemic signs and symptoms**	As above, plus short course of systemic corticosteroids (methylprednisolone 1 mg/kg daily for 3 days, then tapered over 3 more days)

Table 7. Prophylactic measures

Causative Agent	Prophylaxis
■ **Bedbugs**	Treat room with insecticides; use repellents
■ **Fleas**	Treat room with insecticides; use repellents; treat affected pets
■ **Bees and wasps**	Wear appropriate clothing; do not walk on grass barefoot; take care when eating outdoors; if systemic reaction occurs, allergy set and hyposensitization
■ **Mosquitoes and flies**	Wear appropriate clothing; use repellents; perhaps prophylactic antihistamines
■ **Trombidiosis**	Avoid meadows and shrubs; use repellents
■ **Cheyletiella**	Treat affected animals; remove them from household until cleared
■ **Chicken, bird mites**	Treat affected animals; clean and disinfect cages; with asthma, prick testing and specific IgE

Therapy

The therapeutic approach depends on the number and severity of the bites, as shown in Table 6. In the case of an anaphylactic reaction, the patient should carry an emergency kit when outdoors. For children, the usual components are an antihistamine and a corticosteroid, both in liquid form, and a bronchodilator as an inhalant. Individuals who have a systemic reaction to hymenoptera toxin should be desensitized, as about 90% respond well.

Therapy should also include the prophylactic measures outlined in Table 7 and the individual chapters on lice, ticks and scabies. Every effort should be made to avoid repeated exposure for the patient and those in the same environment. The best insect repellents are those containing DEET (N,N-diethyl-3-methylbenzamide); the many natural agents popular in Germany are less effective than DEET and also much shorter lasting. In general, the higher the concentration of DEET, the better, although with children we tend to favor those products in the lower concentration ranges. Children who react dramatically to certain arthropod assaults and will be at risk, as on a camping trip, may do well to take a prophylactic long-acting non-sedating antihistamine such as cetirizine or loratadine. Protective clothing is also sensible.

References

Alexander J.O.: Arthropods in human skin. Springer, Berlin (1984)

Gouck, H.K.: Protection from ticks, fleas, chiggers and leeches. Archives of Dermatology 93:112–113 (1966)

Hurwitz S.: Insect bites and parasitic infestations, S. 405–431. In: Clinical pediatric dermatology, 2nd ed. (1993)

Karppinen A., Kautiainen H., Reunala T., Petman L., Reunala T., Brummer-Korvenkontio H.: Loratadine in the treatment of moscito-bite-sensitive children. Allergy 55:668–671 (2000)

Karppinen A., Petman L., Jeukunen A., Kautiainen H., Vaalasti A., Reunala T.: Treatment of moscito bites with ebastine: a field trial. Acta Dermato-Venereologica 80:114–116 (2000)

Valentine M.D., Schuberth K.C., Kagey-Sobotka A.: The value of immunotherapy with venom in children with allergy to insect stings. New England Journal of Medicine 323:1601–1603

Chapter 4 Atopic Dermatitis

A. Heidelberger, D. Abeck

Epidemiology

Atopic dermatitis is by far the most common type of dermatitis and a major problem in pediatric populations. Synonyms for the disease include atopic eczema and neurodermatitis. Many lay people simply use the term eczema. We equate eczema and dermatitis, and will use exclusively the term dermatitis to reduce confusion. The great socio-economic of atopic dermatitis is demonstrated by the following numbers; in Germany the total costs annual are about 3.5 million €, an average yearly cost of around 2,500 € per patient. The individual and family loss in quality of life has just begun to be quantified with recent studies, but is immense. Most of the patients are children. With an incidence in Germany of between 8 to 16%, atopic dermatitis is the most common skin disease in infancy and childhood. About 60% of the patients show the first signs of their disease during the first year of life. The male: female ratio is about equal.

Pathogenesis

Atopy can be defined as "a familial hypersensitivity of skin and mucous membranes against environmental substances, associated with increased IgE production and/or altered non-specific reactivity". Atopic dermatitis is the skin disorder associated with atopy; its pathogenesis remains confusing. The causes are almost certainly multifactorial. Genetic factors, abnormal responses to environmental allergens and an exaggerated or distorted immune response all seem to be factors. Maternal smoking during pregnancy and nursing appears to raise the risk of atopic dermatitis. In addition, there are a long list of provocation factors, discussed later in the chapter.

Clinical Features

The clinical features of atopic dermatitis vary depending on the stage of the disease (acute or chronic) and the age of the patient. An acute flare is characterized by irregularly bordered erythematous patches with scales, vesicles, weeping, crusting and almost always excoriations (Fig. 7). More chronic lesions show an exaggeration of the skin relief lines known as lichenification (Fig. 8). Pigmentary changes may include pityriasis alba, circumscribed local hypopigmentation, most common on the cheeks and better seen in darker skin individuals. In addition, as patches of atopic dermatitis heal, they may leave behind post-inflammatory hypo- or hyperpigmentation. About 90% of the patients have dry skin because of reduced sebum production or flow. Other typical signs of atopic dermatitis include prominent infraorbital folds (Dennie-Morgan lines), lateral thinning of the eyebrows (Hertoghe sign), white dermographism and hyperlinear palms (ichthyosis hand). Keratosis pilaris, plugging of the hair follicles primarily on the triceps area, is more common in atopic patients; it may also been seen on the thighs and cheeks.

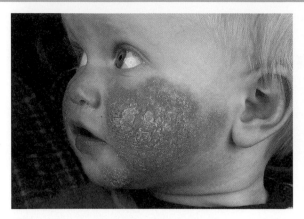

Fig. 7. Atopic dermatitis. The cheeks and chin show diffuse irregular erythema with yellow scales and crusts.

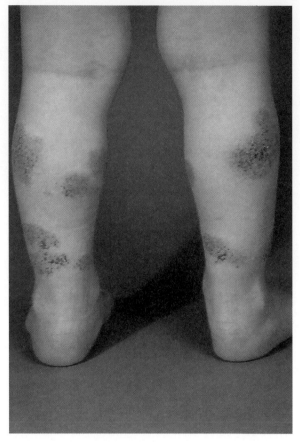

Fig. 9. Atopic dermatitis. In the nummular variant, there are coin-shaped, minimally inflamed erythematous patches and plaques with scale.

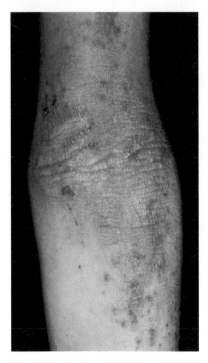

Fig. 8. Atopic dermatitis. Antecubital fossa showing typical erythema, lichenification and excoriations.

There are also a number of clinical variants of atopic dermatitis. Some, such as cheilitis (lip "dermatitis") and foot dermatitis, are covered separately at the end of this section. Another is nummular (coin-shaped) atopic dermatitis (Fig. 9), most common in the first three years of life and in our experience associated with less severe disease. Dys-

hidrotic hand and foot dermatitis may also be a manifestation of atopic dermatitis. Two serious complications of atopic dermatitis which often result in hospitalization are secondary bacterial infections, usually caused by *Staphylococcus aureus* (impetiginized atopic dermatitis), and disseminated herpes simplex virus infections (eczema herpeticum).

Symptoms

The hallmark symptom of atopic dermatitis is pruritus, often intense and unrelenting. In acute flares of disease, it is almost impossible for the patient to control their scratching.

Diagnosis

The diagnosis of atopic dermatitis is usually clinical. Additional measures may include determination of total IgE; identification of allergen-specific IgE via RAST; allergy testing such as prick or atopy patch testing; and an oral provocation challenge for possible food allergies. In some instances bacterial or viral cultures may be needed.

While these measures are usually sufficient for the management of the individual patient, one must be aware that there is still no gold standard for the absolute diagnosis of atopic dermatitis. This is reflected throughout the literature as one attempts to understand incidence and prevalence, or the association of atopic dermatitis with other diseases.

The severity of atopic dermatitis can be quantified with a number of scoring systems. This allows one to better assess the response to therapy and is an essential part of all clinical intervention assessments. We prefer the SCORAD (Severity Scoring of Atopic Dermatitis) index.

Differential Diagnosis

The differential diagnostic considerations for atopic dermatitis are shown in Table 8.

Therapy

The key to the successful management of atopic dermatitis is a multi-faceted approach involving the patient, parents and a wide variety of health professionals with a single physician (usually a dermatologist or pediatrician) heading the effort. In our clinic, we attempt to involve psychologists, dietitians and social workers, as well as seeking appropriate consultation from colleagues.

It has become abundantly clear that simply treating acute flares is not an appropriate approach. Instead, the patient must have a regimen to follow during relatively disease-

Table 8. Differential diagnosis of atopic dermatitis

Diagnosis	Distinguishing Features
■ Seborrheic dermatitis	Usually appears in the first weeks of life, often in the diaper region; moist scales with only minimal pruritus
■ Psoriasis	Usually involves the diaper region (overlap with seborrheic dermatitis) as well as hands; coarse thick scales; often a family history of psoriasis
■ Tinea	Face usually spared; peripheral erythema and scale with positive KOH and culture
■ Scabies	Typically involves hands and feet with sparing of typical sites for atopic dermatitis; papules and papulo-vesicles; often possible to identify *Sarcoptes scabiei*

free intervals and must be instructed in avoiding provocation factors (Table 9). In Germany, this approach is made easier because the manufacturers of virtually all of the widely used topical anti-inflammatory agents (i.e., corticosteroids) also provide the corresponding vehicle free of active ingredients for interval therapy. This approach has high patient acceptance, as they are then using the "same" product in a customized fashion.

■ **Adjuvant Topical Therapy.** Almost all atopic dermatitis patients have dry skin with an impaired epidermal barrier function. The goal is to help restore this barrier through appropriate skin care, adjusted for the activity of their disease and the season of the year. For example, marked occlusion from ointments or pastes must be avoided during warm months as it often leads to increased pruritus; on the other hand, in the winter months many individuals prefer to greasy their skin. It is generally simplest to ask the child and/or parents what seems to work best – ointments or creams and lotions. One can simply ask "Do you do better with something greasy or something that rubs in?" If the child does not like the feel or

Table 9. Therapeutic strategy for atopic dermatitis

1. Maintenance or basic therapy
■ Topical therapy with creams, lotions or emollient ointments
 – products with no active ingredients (i.e., no corticosteroids)
 – addition of moisturizing factors (urea, lactic acid)
 – bath oils (spreading type preferred)

2. Anti-inflammatory therapy of flares
■ Topical
 – corticosteroids
 – perhaps combined with wet compresses
 – antiseptics or dyes
■ Systemic
 – antihistamines
 – antibiotics

3. Avoidance of provocation factors

4. Patient education: the goal is "self-management", not "patient management"

smell of a product, forget it! In addition, be aware that the daily struggles over skin treatment can become a central power struggle between the affected child and the parents, often increasing the family stress level.

The following principles should be followed:

■ The entire body should be treated with the selected maintenance product twice daily.

■ Ointments should be avoided on the face, in intertriginous regions, and during warm months.

■ New products should be tested for a few days on a localized site, usually the flexural surface of the forearm, before being applied to the entire body.

■ Products containing urea are very useful for maintaining skin moisture but burn for a few minutes after application (stinging effect). Once this can be explained to a child, acceptance is no problem. We tend not to employ urea-containing products in children less than 5 years of age.

■ Allergic contact dermatitis is uncommon in children. Often when the patient no longer tolerates a skin care product, an allergy is suspected. If a different prod-

uct is used for about two weeks, the original product can then be used again in virtually all cases.

■ Bath oils may also be very helpful. Most children enjoy bathing and this provides an easy way to further enhance maintenance therapy. There are two basic categories of bath oils – spreading and emulsion. The former remains on the surface of the water and leaves a film on the patient as they leave the tub. We prefer this method and usually employ an almond oil or omega-fatty-acid-based product. We find there is greater patient acceptance and better skin lubrication. The emulsion oils dissolve in the bath water, coating the tub as well as the patient and are clinically less effective. Mild soaps or syndets should be used but only to cleanse dirty areas. Bubble baths must be avoided. Following bathing, the patient should pat dry and reapply the basic care product.

■ **Anti-inflammatory Treatment of Flares.** One of the classic clinical features of atopic dermatitis is rapid flaring. The patient and parents must be in a position to immediately institute anti-inflammatory measures to bring the disease again under control, rather than allowing it to progress. The goal is always rapid control and a return to maintenance therapy.

■ **Topical Corticosteroids.** Topical corticosteroids remain the most effective anti-inflammatory agents available for atopic dermatitis. There are a variety of newer products available with an improved benefit to risk ratio. Included in this group are the active ingredients prednicarbate, hydrocortisone 17-butyrate, hydrocortisone aceponate, methylprednisolone and mometasone fluorate. In Germany, a significant portion of the population is afraid of corticosteroids in any form and extremely resistant to their use. While there is no question that with long-term use or inappropriate choice of agents, the whole range of corticosteroid side effects (including purpura, striae, telangiectases, acne, hirsutism and even systemic effects) can be seen, in most instances the problems associated with untreated atopic dermatitis far outweigh the risks associated with appropriate use of corticosteroids. One must patiently try to convince parents of this fact; often the task is impossible and the child suffers.

There are two general approaches to the short-term use of topical corticosteroids – the step method and the interval method. In the step method, one replaces the initially more potent agent with either a lower concentration of the same active ingredient or a weaker agent. We prefer the interval method, in which the same product is used for the entire regimen, but the frequency of application is sharply reduced. For example, during a flare the product can be applied once daily, and then later, every other day or every third day. We often have patients apply the corticosteroid product only once a week for many months; this is generally effective and has absolutely no risk of side effects. Since the pruritus is usually worse at night, we usually recommend using the corticosteroid product in the evening. If possible, one should avoid using corticosteroids on the face or genitalia. If it is absolutely necessary, then only a hydrocortisone cream or ointment should be chosen.

■ **Topical Immunomodulatory Agents.** The macrolides tacrolimus (Protopic®) and pimecrolimus (Elidel®) have recently been introduced as topical agents and are gradually becoming available worldwide. Both function in a manner similar to cyclosporine A in that they block the transcription of pro-inflammatory cytokine genes. The topical products have been tested in adults and children with atopic dermatitis and are about as effective as mid-potency topical corticosteroids. They have none of the associated corticosteroid side effects, such as atrophy, and there is no suggestion at this point of other serious long-term problems. Since they are immunomodulators, there is possible concern about the induction of cutaneous tumors, especially if their use is combined (inappropriately) with ultraviolet irradiation. Continuing studies will provide further information about long-term safety.

One special problem with tacrolimus is intense burning upon application; this usually improves after a few days of treatment and is only occasionally a reason for stopping therapy, but may limit the product's use in smaller children. This problem has not been seen with pimecrolimus. Both agents are expensive, with the cost of a 50 g tube well over 100 €; this will probably limit their application more than any scientific considerations. The major indications currently are facial, genital or intertriginous atopic dermatitis that fails to respond to intermittent low-potency corticosteroids, as well as rare refractory cases of widespread disease where in the past oral cyclosporine A was employed.

■ **Other Anti-Inflammatory agents.** As a result of the corticosteroid phobia in Germany, a wide variety of other anti-inflammatory products are frequently prescribed. None are more effective than 1% hydrocortisone cream. Included in the group are bufexamac (a non-steroidal anti-inflammatory drug) cream, a variety of phytopharmaceuticals (for example, witch hazel or liquorice), coal tars and shale tars (ichthyol).

Probably the most widely prescribed member of this group is bufexamac. We find it to have a very minimal anti-inflammatory action. In recent years, there have been a number of reports of allergic contact dermatitis to bufexamac. Although the risk is probably quite small when one considers how often it is prescribed, if allergic contact dermatitis develops, it can be particularly difficult to identify and severe in those with atopic dermatitis. Often it continues to progress once the bufexamac has been stopped. In some instances, a short burst of systemic corticosteroids (methylprednisolone 0.5 mg/kg for 3 days and then 0.25 mg/kg for another 3 days) is needed to quiet down the

Atopic Dermatitis

reaction. For these reasons we cannot recommend topical bufexamac.

The other agents are equally ineffective. In addition, there are concerns about the carcinogenicity of tars, which are no longer available in many European countries. We do occasionally employ ichthyol products in children. Its objectionable smell, staining of skin, clothing and bedding, and lack of effectiveness make its use extremely limited.

■ **Topical Antimicrobial Agents.** Weeping areas of atopic dermatitis often have larger numbers of *Staphylococcus aureus*. The traditional treatment for such lesions has been dye solutions, which are both astringent and antimicrobial. For example gentian violet has a good effect against Gram-positive organisms. We still use 0.25% aqueous gentian violet (reduced to 0.1% on mucosa and transitional zones) in children, usually applying it once or on occasion twice daily. The risks of disturbed wound healing or necrosis are non-existent with this concentration and regimen. While the discoloration of the child and their environment does occur, it usually disturbs the parents and health care personnel far more than the patient.

When larger areas must be treated, we generally use the antiseptics triclosan (1–2%) or chlorhexidine gluconate (1%). Either can be mixed with the patient's maintenance product and provide good coverage against Gram-positive cocci. In contrast, the old favorite clioquinol (Vioform®) is only minimally effective against the same bacteria. We no longer use it for widespread disease because of the risks of systemic absorption and allergic contact dermatitis.

■ **Systemic Antibiotics.** Patients with widespread weeping atopic dermatitis can be assumed to be infected with *Staphylococcus aureus*. The use of systemic antibiotics usually brings prompt improvement. In most western lands, many strains of *Staphylococcus aureus* are resistant to erythromycin, so a first generation cephalosporin or a penicillinase-resistant penicillin should be chosen. If the patient is allergic to penicillin, clindamycin is probably the best choice.

■ **Antipruritic Therapy with Antihistamines.** Antihistamines may offer a small amount of relief from the pruritus associated with flares of atopic dermatitis (see Appendix). In general, sedating H1 antihistamines should be used, with careful attention to age-specific guidelines. We usually use doxylamine succinate, dimethindene maleate or hydroxyzine. It usually suffices to prescribe the agents only in the evening. Although the official recommendation is to taper the medications following long-term use, practical problems with withdrawal do not exist. A paradoxical reaction can occur in some children who become hyperactive rather than sedated.

Non-sedating antihistamines such as loratadine or cetirizine, and their newer modifications descarboethoxyloratidine or levocetirizine dihydrochloride, are often prescribed for atopic dermatitis but there is no good evidence for their effectiveness and we have been disappointed. Topical antihistamines should be avoided for long-term use, as the incidence of allergic contact dermatitis is disturbingly high.

■ **Supportive Measures.** Another favorite trick of ours is the use of "wet pajamas" in the treatment of exacerbated atopic dermatitis. While this approach was initially used for in-patients, it can also be adapted for home use. Our protocol is shown in Table 10. Usually after just a few days there is such dramatic improvement that maintenance therapy can be resumed.

Special cotton pajamas (for example, Lotties® Neurodermatitis Overall) are available which cover the entire body, including the hands and feet, leaving only the head exposed. They effectively prevent a child from doing any damage by scratching. Another innovative fabric is coated with silver on the inner surface (Padycare®). The silver coating has an antibacterial effect, especially against *Staphylococcus aureus*, and in clinical studies, patients using these pajamas do better

Table 10. Application of wet compresses

1. Tubular dressings (Tubifast®) are cut for the trunk, arms and legs
2. Application of the non-medicated basic product
3. Dressings are moistened with lukewarm water or a 0.5% chlorhexidine aqueous solution
4. Application of the moist dressings to the skin
5. Application of a second dry set of dressings
6. Underlying dressings re-moistened every 3 hours
7. At noon, re-application of the basic product and re-application of dressings
8. In the evening, bathing using a bath oil
9. Re-application of the basic product
10. For overnight, re-application of moist dressings
11. *For severe disease, a corticosteroid can be used instead of the maintenance product*

Table 11. Major provocation factors for atopic dermatitis

■ **Non-specific factors (general reaction patterns)**
- irritants
  hard water, clothing, bathing habits
- immune stimulation
  infections, immunizations
- microbial colonization of skin
  Staphylococcus aureus, herpes simplex virus or *Pityrosporum ovale*
- climate
  variations in climate, photosensitivity
- emotional factors and stress

■ **Specific factors (individual reaction patterns)**
- allergies
  food, house dust mites, animal hairs, pollens
- contact allergies
- pseudoallergies (idiosyncratic and intolerance reactions)
  preservatives or citrus fruits

than those in ordinary cotton pajamas. In some instances, the insurance companies will help pay for such special clothing.

Specialized rehabilitation clinics for atopic dermatitis are available in Europe; many are on the sea shore or in the higher mountains such as Davos, Switzerland. It is unclear if the change in environment, or if specific features of the site (fewer allergens, more or different sunlight), play the most important role. Most of the centers have special programs for children, trying to teach the child and hopefully their family to manage the disease, rather than just providing 3–6 weeks of relief.

■ **Provocation Factors.** Identifying and then avoiding provocation factors is another important aspect of treating atopic dermatitis. The major factors are shown in Table 11.

Because of their disturbed barrier function, patients with atopic dermatitis are in general more susceptible to skin irritation, whatever the source – soap, frequent water contact, wool, synthetic fabrics, sweating. They also react differently to challenges to their immune system (infections, bacterial colonization, immunizations) and to emotional stresses.

Hypersensitivity to specific allergens can be identified by skin tests (prick tests and patch tests), blood tests (RAST) and direct challenge (provocation testing). The atopy patch test procedure will soon be commercially available and should expand the possibilities for allergy evaluation.

The role of food allergies in atopic dermatitis is generally overestimated. Relevant food allergies are found in 10–20% of patients, almost exclusively in infants and small children who usually have significant skin disease. The gold standard for diagnosing a food allergy is a double-blind, placebo-controlled oral challenge test. If this is positive, then the child should avoid the relevant foods. It is important that the child not avoid a wide range of foods because such an approach is rarely justified and can lead to nutritional disturbances. The child should be re-challenged occasionally to document the need for further avoidance.

Some patients notice that their atopic dermatitis worsens after exposure to tree, grass and weed pollens, animal hairs or house dust mites. If prick and serologic testing confirms the allergy, then avoidance measures should be undertaken. For animal hair allergies, the approach is usually simple. In the case of house dust mites, special coverings for mattresses, pillows and bedding, frequent washing of bedding, frequent vacuum cleaning and elimination of carpets and upholstered furniture may be helpful. In the case of pollen allergies, the situation is more difficult.

■ **Immunizations.** Children with atopic dermatitis, even with widespread skin disease, should receive the standard immunization series. Occasionally their skin disease may flare with an immunization, but this can be easily treated. Children should not be treated during an acute flare or if they are receiving immunosuppressive therapy (such as systemic corticosteroids). The parents must understand that the risks to the child and to society are greater when immunizations are avoided. Of course, they must avoid vaccination with vaccinia and exposure to others who have received this vaccination; this caution may become important as the USA is reconsidering the use of smallpox vaccinations for some groups.

■ **Social Aspects.** The entire health care team should be sensitive to the family situation and the many stresses which can develop when one or more children have atopic dermatitis. The goal is to avoid strained parent-child, especially mother-child, relationships which can have long-term disastrous effects. Adjuvant psychological aid should be enlisted whenever there is a hint of home problems.

Once again, the only successful therapy regimen is one which enlists the efforts of the affected child and his family. The patients should be actively trained to learn about their disease and how they can take responsibility for its management, rather than just passively accepting what comes along. The goal is to make each patient an expert in their disease. Said in other words, we often tell patients "It doesn't matter how good a doctor I am; all that matters is how smart a patient (or parent) you are." While this may be a bit exaggerated and ego-damaging, it is close to the truth.

References

Abeck, D., Ring J. (eds) Atopisches Ekzem im Kindesalter. Das zeitgemäße Management. Steinkopff (2002)

Abeck D., Strom K.: Optimal management of atopic dermatitis. American Journal of Clinical Dermatology 1:41–46 (2000)

Abeck D., Mempel M.: Kutane *Staphylococcus aureus*-Besiedelung des atopischen Ekzems. Mechanismen, pathophysiologische Bedeutung und therapeutische Konsequenzen. Hautarzt 49:902–906 (1998)

Abeck D., Cremer H., Pflugshaupt C.: Stadienorientierte Auswahl dermatologischer Grundlagen ("Vehikel") bei der ärztlichen Therapie des atopischen Ekzems. pädiatrische praxis 52:113–121 (1997)

Bieber T., Leung D.Y.M. (eds) Atopic dermatitis. Marcel Dekker, New York, Basel (2002)

Cremer H.: Children with "sensitive" skin. The role of skin irritation in the development of atopic eczema. European Journal of Pediatric Dermatology 3:13–20 (1993)

Defaie F., Abeck D., Brockow K., Vieluf D., Hamm M., Behr-Völtzer C., Ring J.: Konzept einer altersabhängigen Basis- und Aufbaudiät für Säuglinge und Kleinkinder mit nahrungsmittelassoziiertem atopischem Ekzem. Allergo Journal 5:231–235 (1996)

European TASK Force on Atopic Dermatitits. Severity scoring of atopic dermatitis: the SCORAD index. Dermatology 186:23–31 (1993)

Griese M.: Differentialdiagnose und Behandlung des atopischen Ekzems im Kindes- und Jugendalter. Monatsschrift für Kinderheilkunde 145:73–84 (1997)

Höger P.H.: Topische Antibiotika und Antiseptika. Agentien, Spektren und Nebenwirkungen. Hautarzt 49:331–347 (1998)

Kang S., Lucky A.W., Pariser D., Lawrence I., Hanifin J.M.: Long-term safety and efficacy of tacrolimus ointment for the treatment of atopic dermatitis in children. Journal of the American Academy of Dermatology 44:S58–64 (2001)

Klein P.A., Clark R.A.F.: An evidence-based review of the efficacy of antihistamines in relieving pruritus in atopic dermatitis. Archives of Dermatology 135:1522–1525 (1999)

Leung D.Y.M.: Atopic dermatitis: new insights and opportunities for therapeutic intervention. Journal of Allergy and Clinical Immunology 105:860–876 (2000)

Mallon E., Powell S., Bridgman A.: Wet-wrap dressings for the treatment of atopic eczema in the community. Journal of Dermatological Treatment 5:97–98 (1994)

Niedner R.: Kortikoide in der Dermatologie. UNI-MED, Bremen (1998)

Paller A., Eichenfield L. F., Leung D. Y. M., Stewart D., Appell M.: A 12-week study of tacrolimus ointment for the treatment of atopic dermatitis in pediatric patients. Journal of the American Academy of Dermatology 44:S47–57 (2001)

Ring J., Abeck D.: Vom "Patienten-Management" zum "Selbst-Management": Prävention durch Schulung bei atopischem Ekzem (Neurodermitis). S. 32–41. In: v. Stünzner W., Giesler M. (Hrsg.) Prävention allergischer Erkrankungen im Kindes- und Jugendalter. Kohlhammer, Stuttgart (1996)

Van Leent E. J. M., Graber M., Thurston M., Wagenaar A., Spuls P. I., Bos J. D.: Effectiveness of the ascomycin macrolactam SDZ ASM 981 in the topical treatment of atopic dermatitis. Archives of Dermatology 134:805–809 (1998)

Williams H. C.: Atopic Dermatitis. The Epidemiology, Causes and Prevention of Atopic Eczema. Cambridge University Press (2000)

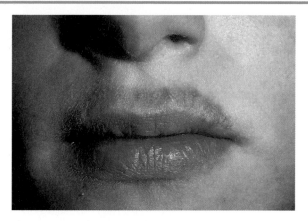

Fig. 10. Atopic dermatitis. Lick cheilitis with typical erythema and modest scaling of the perioral skin where the child has licked or chewed their often dry lips.

Atopic Cheilitis

C. Schnopp

Epidemiology

While no exact numbers for the prevalence of atopic cheilitis are available, it is a common clinical problem.

Pathogenesis

Atopic cheilitis is also known in German as lick cheilitis. It is a common type of cumulative-toxic (chronic irritant) dermatitis. Many children with atopic dermatitis suffer from dry, often cracked lips (cheilitis sicca). In our climatic zone, this is much more common in winter. The patient responds to the problem by licking (usually upper lip) or chewing (usually lower lip) and the resultant irritation makes the problem worse, leading to repeated licking and a vicious circle evolves. In infants using a pacifier, the problem may be limited to the area in contact with the moist object. Children without atopic dermatitis may develop similar changes but in our practice the problem is much more common in those with atopy.

Clinical Features

The perioral skin extending up to the vermilion border is erythematous, dry and has fine scales. The affected skin has been compared to parchment. The transition to normal skin is usually sharp. There may be associated angular cheilitis (perlèche) or excoriations (Fig. 10). The lips themselves are usually dry and cracked (cheilitis sicca). The main complications are secondary impetiginization and less often herpes simplex virus infections.

Symptoms

True pruritus, so typical for atopic dermatitis, does not often affect the lips. The feeling is usually one of tightness or dryness. Whatever name is attached, the patient is bothered enough that they respond.

Diagnosis

The diagnosis is clinical. Often the patient denies licking and other manipulation, but upon observation for a few minutes or in

Atopic Dermatitis

Table 12. Differential diagnosis of atopic cheilitis

Diagnosis	Distinguishing Features
■ **Perioral dermatitis**	Usually succulent papules and erythema, not extending to the vermilion border (Grenz zone) with only occasional dermatitis; often perinasal or periocular changes
■ **Herpes labialis**	Grouped blisters with erosions and crusts; lesions usually not flat
■ **Acrodermatitis enteropathica**	Marked erythema, crusting and scale perioral, but also perinasal, about genitalia; usually associated with malnutrition and other systemic problems
■ **Allergic contact dermatitis**	Skin changes irregularly bordered and quite pruritic; positive patch testing

Table 13. Treatment of lick cheilitis

■ **During the day**	Repeated application of ointment or lip balm
■ **Evenings**	Protect with 1% chlorhexidine or 5% almond oil in soft zinc paste
■ **Marked inflammation**	Corticosteroid emollient cream or ointment in the evening for 3–5 nights

References

Higgins E., duVivier A. (eds.) Skin diseases in childhood and adolescence, pp. 51–52. Blackwell, Oxford (1996)

the waiting room, they will almost always reflexively lick their lips.

Differential Diagnosis

The differential diagnostic considerations are summarized in Table 12.

Therapy

During the day, the lips and adjacent skin should be frequently lubricated. One can sometimes convince the patient to use an emollient ointment or lip balm rather than licking. We often compound a lip ointment as follows:

■ Rx_

dexpanthenol ointment
unguentum molle aa ad 30.0 g

At night a protective paste can be employed. Topical corticosteroids only make sense if the skin is markedly inflamed; we then suggest applying a mid-potency ointment only in the evening for several nights. In some instances, psychological help may be needed to enable the patient to give up or minimize the habit of lip licking.

Foot Dermatitis in Atopic Patients

H. Fesq

Epidemiology

Foot dermatitis is most common in children between 8 and 14 years of age. Exact figures for the prevalence are not available. Childhood foot dermatitis is seen most commonly in atopic individuals but is surely not limited to this group. There are two clinically different conditions which may overlap – atopic winter feet and atopic foot dermatitis.

Pathogenesis

Trigger factors for atopic winter feet include improper foot hygiene, irritation and the wearing of shoes which are more occlusive (such as many athletic shoes and most shoes manufactured from synthetic products). In parts of North America, the problem is known as snowmobile boot syndrome, since it is so much more common in winter when children are wearing totally occlusive shoes or boots. Atopic foot dermatitis may arise on this background or as part of severe atopic dermatitis. It is often complicated by allergic contact dermatitis.

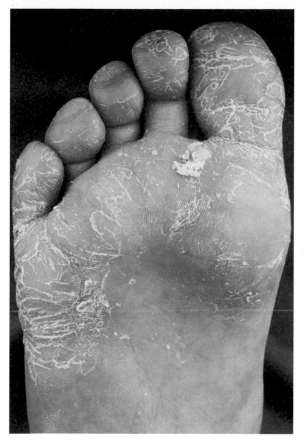

Fig. 11. Atopic winter foot. Erythema and scaling limited to sole of foot.

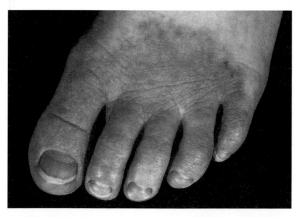

Fig. 12. Atopic foot dermatitis. Chronic diffuse erythematous patch with prominent skin markings involving dorsum of foot.

Clinical Features

The classic features of atopic winter feet are bilateral symmetry and almost exclusive plantar involvement (Fig. 11). In contrast, atopic foot dermatitis may be unilateral, presenting with erythema and scaling of the skin of the distal dorsal foot, usually including the toes and often extended to the most distal ventral surface (Fig. 12). Excoriations may be found and cracking (fissures or rhagades) are common and frequently painful.

Symptoms

Atopic winter feet are usually asymptomatic. Atopic foot dermatitis may be pruritic or painful, depending on the severity of the problem.

Differential Diagnosis

The differential diagnostic considerations are listed in Table 14.

Table 14. Differential diagnosis of atopic foot dermatitis

Diagnosis	Distinguishing Features
■ **Tinea pedum**	Scales are more prominent at periphery of lesion; rarely symmetrical; less pruritic; KOH examination and culture positive
■ **Allergic contact dermatitis**	Often vesicles or blisters; more likely to be ventral and if caused by shoe products symmetrical; patch testing positive

Atopic Dermatitis

Therapy

Intensive maintenance care is most important, and usually all that is necessary for atopic winter feet. Compounds containing urea or lactic acid seem especially valuable.

Table 15. Treatment of atopic foot dermatitis

■ **Initial (day 1–7)**	Urea-containing cream several times daily; mid-potency topical corticosteroid at night if inflamed
■ **Maintenance**	Continue urea-containing product; 10% almond oil in soft zinc paste or 5% ichthyol in soft zinc paste at night; topical corticosteroid 1–2 × weekly

For maintenance therapy, we often employ pastes containing ichthyol (Table 15). Patients should be encouraged to go barefoot as much as possible or to wear sandals. They should avoid occlusive shoes. When dermatitis is present, topical corticosteroids are usually needed at least briefly.

References

Jones S.K., English J.S.C., Forsyth A., Mackie R.M.: Juvenile plantar dermatosis – an 8 year follow-up of 102 patients. Clinical and Experimental Dermatology 12:5–7 (1987)

CHAPTER 5

Burns and Sunburn

B. Heidtmann, O. Brandt

Burns

Epidemiology

Burns are the third most common accident involving children in Germany. They follow only traffic accidents and drownings. There are correlations between the type of burn, the age of the patient and the socioeconomic status.

In children up to 3 years of age, scaldings with hot water are the most common burns. They may occur when a child pulls a pot from the stove, in which case the face, neck, chest and arms are involved. Such burns reflect a lack of supervision. More serious are immersion burns when bath water is too hot for the child. Here the burns involve the legs, buttocks and lower trunk and usually have a sharp border. Child abuse should be suspected in such cases.

Burns in older children and teenagers usually result from playing with open fires. Once again, the hands, face and upper trunk are most often affected. The number of burns is greater in the summer as outdoor grilling provides an easy exposure to flammable materials.

Pathogenesis

A temperature of $45°C$ on the skin is sufficient to cause an erythema; $55°C$ can produce blisters and when $60°C$ is exceeded, necrosis occurs because of denaturation and coagulation of proteins. The actual physical insult is followed by the release of mediators from the skin, producing erythema, warmth, swelling, pain and limiting function. The edema results from the leakage of proteins, electrolytes and water through capillaries into the extravascular space.

Clinical Features

Burns are usually divided clinically into 4 stages or degrees:
- *First-degree burn* – damage to the upper layers of the epidermis with hyperemia, erythema and swelling; painful; heals without scarring.

- *Second-degree burn*
Grade 2a – damage to the epidermis with subepidermal blister; painful; heals without scarring (Fig. 13).
Grade 2b – subepidermal blister with damage to epidermis, dermis and sometimes adnexal structures; dermis below the blister appears white; painful; heals with scarring.

- *Third-degree burn* – gray-white skin, usually dry, with necrotic crusts and debris; damage of the entire skin into the subcutaneous tissue, with destruction of nerve endings; deeper lying structures such as tendons, muscles and bones may be affected; painless; healing with marked scar formation, often hypertrophic scars or keloids. While a deep burn is itself not painful, the patient is always in pain with less severe burns at the periphery of the deeper injury.

It is difficult to assess the depth of a burn at first inspection. When burned tissue is

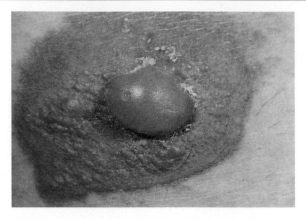

Fig. 13. Second-degree burn. Large blister with clear fluid, as well as tiny confluent blisters starting in the rest of the erythematous burn site.

not adequately cooled, there may be what has been called "after burning". This means that the heat is kept in the tissue and becomes transmitted to adjacent parts of the burned skin causing further damage. Often the damage becomes more apparent first several hours or days later, so that only then can the true depth be assessed.

The extent of burns is traditionally determined by the well-known "Rule of Nines". However, for assessing burns in newborns and infants where the body proportions are different, the palmar surface of the patient's hand, including the fingers, accounts for about 1% of the skin surface.

Symptoms

The main symptom is pain. Paradoxically, it is a "good" sign as it suggests there is no full-thickness damage. Some patients with intact tense blisters may also find these uncomfortable.

Diagnosis

The diagnosis is not difficult in most cases. One must just look and ask the patient or the parents. Two cautions – never forget the possibility of child abuse leading to a scald or burn. Equally important, children with

staphylococcal scalded skin syndrome may also be erroneously diagnosed as burned and not receive the appropriate therapy. Differential diagnosis is further complicated by the possibility of secondary infection with *Staphylococcus aureus*. If there is increasing erythema, blistering or exfoliation, appropriate bacterial studies should be performed. Rapid testing for staphylococcal exfoliative toxins will be available soon, making it much easier to exclude primary and secondary staphylococcal infections.

Therapy

The therapy of burns is complex and most often handled in specialized centers. In addition, many other burns are treated in hospitals so the dermatologist or pediatrician in practice is likely to be confronted primarily with first-degree and superficial second-degree burns. Nonetheless, we present our experience with burns from the perspective of a pediatric dermatology referral clinic with the opportunity to hospitalize patients.

The essential initial step in treating a burn is cooling after the clothing has been removed. This should be started as a emergency procedure by the first person confronted with the burn. Water or normal saline solution can be poured over the burn, or the burn immersed; this should be done for at least 30 minutes. If the cooling cannot be continued as the patient is brought to the doctor, then the burn should be covered with a non-adherent dressing such as Metalline® Foil.

The rest of the therapeutic approach depends on the depth of the wounds. Second- and third-degree burns require tetanus booster shot (or complete immunization in rare cases).

■ First-degree Burns

In the case of first-degree burns, moist compresses are used for several hours. Then either 5% polidocanol in a water-based lotion (or lotio alba aqueosa) or a mid-potency corticosteroid cream or lotion can be applied t.i.d.-q.i.d. for several days. The patient should be re-examined after 24 hours and the dressing changed. After this, most patients can be cared for by their parents.

Acetaminophen suppositories or liquid are usually sufficient for pain relief. The dosage is 125 mg for those <10 kg; 250 mg, <25 kg; and 500 mg for patients >25 kg. The dose can be repeated every six hours.

Aspirin is an excellent analgesic for burn patients. It not only offers pain relief, but also blocks the prostaglandin cascade, thus, reducing the erythema and edema. Aspirin should not be used in children under 15 years of age because of the risk of Reye syndrome (acute encephalopathy and toxic liver degeneration). An absolute contraindication to the use of aspirin in children is a glucose-6-phosphate-dehydrogenase (G6PD) deficiency.

■ Second- and Third-degree Burns

Patients with deep second-degree and third-degree burns usually require hospitalization. The major local measures prior to admission are cooling and covering with a sterile dressing. We view the following as absolute indications for admission to a burn unit:

■ Infants less than 12 months of age, regardless of the extent of the burn, as both analgesia and fluid replacement are difficult in this age group

■ Children in whom there is suspicion of inhalation burns

■ Second- or third-degree burns involving more than 10% of body surface

■ Burns involving face, hands, feet or anogenital region

■ Electric burns, because of the risk of cardiac rhythm disturbances within the first 24–48 hours.

The intact blisters in superficial second-degree burns may feel tense and cause discomfort. The blister should be drained through a small puncture, so that the intact blister roof is retained as a natural dressing. The burn is much more painful if the blister is denuded.

Topical measures must be adjusted to the stage of the burn. Weeping surfaces should be covered with a non-adherent but adsorbent dressing which can then be fixed in place with a loose gauze bandage. Alternative possibilities include silver sulfadiazine cream (Silvadene®, "burn butter") or a gauze impregnated with antibiotics. The dressings should be changed daily. Prior to removal of the dressings, they should be soaked with a sterile saline solution in order to make their removal less painful. The dressings should be continued until wound seepage is only a minor problem. Then silver sulfadiazine cream or a similar product can be used either without dressings or with a lighter wrap. Occasionally enzymes with debriding action such as sutilains (Travase® ointment) can be used to help with debridement. The adjacent areas with only first-degree burns can be treated as above.

More effective pain therapy is usually required. If a child has deep second-degree or third-degree burns, acetaminophen is often not strong enough and either ketamine or opiates are needed (Table 16). The importance of pain relief cannot be overlooked; it is the crux of treating the acute stages of all severe burns.

An adequate intravenous line must be placed. Then 0.1 mg/kg of midazolam is administered, followed by 0.5–0.7 mg/kg of S-ketamine (Ketanest S®). In some extremely anxious children, we first give an intramuscular injection of 0.5 mg/kg of S-ketamine, before attempting to insert the intravenous line. Obviously then, one must reduce the initial intravenous dosage. Two alternatives to ketamine are morphine (0.1 mg/kg) and tramadol (0.5–1.0 mg/kg).

Table 16. Analgesic agents for burn patients

Agent	Dose
■ **S-ketamine**	0.5–1.0 mg/kg (first administer midazolam)
■ **Midazolam**	0.1 mg/kg
■ **Morphine sulfate**	0.1 mg/kg
■ **Tramadol**	0.5–1.0 mg/kg

Volume replacement is another cornerstone in the treatment of burns. The fluid and electrolyte loss is enormous. The usual replacement fluid is Ringer solution or lactated Ringer solution. The usual replacement rate is 20–40 mL/kg/hour. There are complex formulas to assure adequate and correct fluid replacement; we cite these numbers only to show how much fluid may be needed. Plasma expanders are usually not desirable, as they lead to increased wound edema and, thus, hamper the circulatory effort.

Complications

The list of complications following burns is long. The most serious short-term problem is secondary wound infections. The possible bacteria include not only the usual Gram-positive bacteria such as staphylococci and streptococci, but also a wide range of Gram-negative bacteria. The development of resistance is a major problem, as the patients are exposed to a host of anti-microbial agents. The status of the burns should be assessed by frequent wound cultures. Initially a broad spectrum antibiotic such as cefuroxime axetil can be employed and then the agent adjusted depending on the wound culture and sensitivity results.

A feared complication of fires in homes or apartments is the inhalation of smoke and hot gases. This can lead after a delay of many hours to swelling of the mucosa of the upper and lower respiratory tracts. In extreme cases, pulmonary edema with respiratory insufficiency can develop requiring intensive care treatment.

Large or deep burns (more than 10% body surface or third-degree) can lead to marked fluid loss and eventually shock. As the proportion of body surface area to body weight increases, this problem becomes more and more likely.

Circumferential burns on the extremities can lead to edema which is confined by the skin and, thus, compresses the cutaneous vessels, reducing blood flow to the skin which enhances tissue necrosis. Timely relaxing incisions can avoid this complication.

The major late problems with burns are well known to all – scarring and resultant joint contractures. It is essential to start physical therapy as soon as possible if a burn scar extends across a joint. If the pain is too great, ketamine analgesia should be given prior to treatment.

Burn scars tend to be hypertrophic or keloidal. The best prophylaxis against these devastating changes is pressure. Specially tailed elastic compression stockings, sleeves or garments are the best approach. They must be worn for the bulk of the day, ideally for 24 hours. They have a short half-life as they loose their compression with repeated use. In the case of children, if the child is in a rapid growth phase, the garments may have to be re-fitted. They are usually used for 12 months, along with extensive, specialized physical therapy.

For smaller burn scars, usually deep second-degree, a silicone gel sheet can be employed. It can be employed in children of all ages. The self-adherent gel is applied to the area as soon as re-epithelialization has occurred. It is worn around the clock, but the skin and the gel sheet are cleaned gently every 12 hours. Occasionally the skin becomes irritated, but usually therapy can be continued. The sheeting can generally be used for about 2 weeks before it must be replaced. Usually a 3 month period of treatment is required.

Sunburn

Epidemiology

Sunburn is the most common type of acute sunlight-induced skin damage. It is seen in all age groups and at all latitudes. Individuals living where the sun seldom shines have less of a tan and more interest in sun exposure, so they paradoxically have a greater risk of sunburns. The same paradox explains why tourists going to sunny tropical climates or to the mountains to the winter are so likely to be burned, as they try to maximize sun exposure.

The major risk group is those individuals with Type I and II skin. In addition, infants and children are much more susceptible to sunburn. Sunburns in children almost always (>90%) occur under the supervision (or lack thereof) of adults. The body area involved varies considerably with the age group and activity (playing versus sitting in buggy versus lying in the sun). Most sunburn is equivalent to a first-degree burn, although superficial second-degree changes also occur.

The biggest epidemiological problem is that severe sunburns in childhood are a well-established risk factor for the later development of a malignant melanoma. Thus, both dermatologists and pediatricians must work together to convince parents and children to avoid extensive sun exposure.

Pathogenesis

Only a small part of the solar irradiation spectrum causes sunburn. The so-called erythema spectrum or UVB light (290–320 nm) is mainly responsible for sunburns caused by natural light. The exposure damages epidermal keratinocytes which then trigger a prostaglandin-mediated inflammatory reaction. The erythema is the result of the dilatation of vessels in the papillary dermis.

The allegedly safer lower energy UVA irradiation (320–400 nm) can also cause a sunburn, especially when it is delivered via artificial light sources, such as a tanning bed or phototherapy unit. In nature, one receives such a bad UVB burn that no one can stay in the sun long enough to get a true UVA burn. One modifying factor is the use of sunscreens blocking UVB which allow increased levels of UVA to reach the skin. How harmful this is remains controversial. Fortunately, most new sunscreens block both UVB and UVA quite effectively.

Clinical Features

The intensity and clinical course of a sunburn obviously depend on the dose of UVB which the patient receives. In most instances, the patient notices the pain or even erythema, so an intrinsic self-protective mechanism is present preventing severe sunburn. Deeper burns occur only in individuals whose ability to respond is impaired (drugs, alcohol), who use a tanning bed inappropriately or who are unable to move themselves (*infants!*).

A mild sunburn develops 4–6 hours after exposition only in the areas which have been exposed to sunlight. The borders created by clothing, or even patterns on clothing, or improperly applied sunscreen are well known. The erythema reaches its peak at

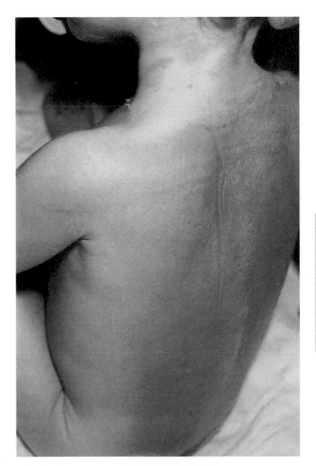

Fig. 14. Sunburn. Sharply bordered flat erythema on the back, upper arms, and thighs without blisters at this point.

Table 17. Skin types (after Fitzpatrick)

Type	Name	Comments	SPF*
I	Celtic	Fair ivory skin; red or blond hair; often blue eyes and freckles; *tans never; burns always*	15–30
II	Fair "Caucasian"	White skin; blond hair; blue or green eyes; occasionally freckles; *tans a little; burns easily*	12–30
III	Dark "Caucasian"	White skin; dirty blond or brown hair; gray or brown eyes; *tans moderately; burns moderately*	8–15
IV	Mediterranean	Beige; dark brown to black hair; brown eyes; *tans easily; burns minimally*	8–12
V	North African, Middle Easterner	Moderate brown skin; black hair; brown eyes; *tans profusely; burns rarely*	6-8
VI	Blacks	Dark brown or black skin; black hair; brown eyes; *tans profusely, burns never*	2–4

*Suggested SPF value of sunscreen for routine use

12–24 hours and resolves by 72–120 hours (Fig. 14). More severe sunburns appear earlier but reach their peak later, often showing maximum changes at 24–48 hours. The erythema is accompanied by edema and blistering. If the burn is mild, the skin does not peel and an increased tan is the result. If the epidermal damage is sufficient, the skin peels, as every reader has certainly observed on themselves. In most cases, only the epidermis peels and regeneration has already occurred, so the new skin is dry.

With fair-skinned children (Type I and II in Table 17) and with high exposure, there may be sufficient irradiation to produce deeper dermal damage leading to scarring. Such wounds do not peel in a dry fashion. Instead, when the blister roof is removed, the wound bed weeps for a number of days, requiring burn care.

Sunburn may also lead to systemic signs and symptoms, including fever, chills, nausea, vomiting, headache and nuchal rigidity. This constellation is known in the USA as "sun poisoning" although no specific toxin has been identified. In Germany, it is described as *Sonnenstich* (sun sting). Most patients have had excessive irradiation to the head, but this is not mandatory. There may be an elevated leukocyte count, elevated hematocrit secondary to dehydration and increased levels of C-reactive protein. In children, the process may have a delayed onset, so a child with a significant sunburn should be checked throughout the night by the parents. There is a gradual transition from sun poisoning to heat stroke with loss of temperature control, seizures and circulatory collapse.

Symptoms

A sunburned child will complain of tenderness, a burning sensation or pain, depending on the severity of the sunburn. Development of the symptoms discussed above reflects a systemic reaction.

Diagnosis

The diagnosis of sunburn is straight-forward. There is no differential diagnosis, but there are a number of photosensitivity diseases which may manifest themselves for the first time following sun exposure, occasionally presenting as a severe sunburn in childhood. Included in this group are xeroderma pigmentosum, some types of porphyria and lupus erythematosus as well as variants of polymorphic light eruption.

Therapy

A mild sunburn can be treated with cold compresses or even wrapping the patient in a moistened towel. Just as with a thermal burn, cooling should be continued for a few hours. Then the area can be treated with 5% polidocanol in zinc oxide lotion or a water-soluble lotion. If the zinc oxide lotion is too drying, a more lubricating vehicle should be chosen. A mid-potency corticosteroid cream or lotion can also be employed. One should not use over-the-counter sunburn products which contain benzocaine. The likelihood of developing an allergic contact dermatitis is high.

The pain should be treated with acetaminophen. The dosage is 125 mg with body weight <10 kg, 250 mg <25 kg; and others 500 mg. The medication can be repeated every 6 hours. In teenagers >15 years of age, 300–600 mg aspirin can replace the acetaminophen, as discussed under burns.

Laboratory experiments have shown that both oral or topical aspirin and topical corticosteroids can block the development of sunburn if they are administered after the UVB exposure but before any erythema develops. While this is true, it is very hard to set into practice. In addition, it is not strategic to offer patients a way to avoid sunburn; they should avoid the sun. On the other hand, following accidental over-exposure in either a tanning bed or in a clinical setting with a phototherapy unit, one can administer systemic aspirin and system corticosteroids in an attempt to abort or minimize the pain and damage.

More severe sunburns are treated just like burns, as discussed in the first half of this section. One should think of tetanus immunization and possible antibiotic coverage.

Preventative Measures

Obviously the message is to avoid sunburn. Parents are responsible for their children, most emphatically for infants who cannot remove themselves from the sun. The maximum solar irradiation occurs around noon and in the early afternoon, so children should not spend this time in the sun. Infants probably should not be exposed to the sun at all, as they lack many protective mechanisms.

Clothing is an effective sun protection mechanism in children. Special clothes are available which are attractive and provide proven protection. Ordinary clothes provide some protection but it is quite difficult to assess how much. For example, a white T-shirt offers little protection, while blue jeans are quite effective, but there is a vast range in between. Often individuals with a patterned garment will receive a sunburn with a pattern, showing the variable protection. One should not forget a hat. Younger children often have sparse hair or short hair cuts and need this additional protection as much as adults.

The third mainstay is sunscreens. We emphasize clothing first, because it is hard to forget your pants and easy to forget your sunscreen. The main criteria for a sunscreen for children is *not* a label saying – sunscreen for children". Instead, one needs an agent which blocks UVB and UVA, has a high sun protection factor (SPF 15–30), is water-resistant, and is free of fragrances and preservatives.

Sunscreens employ both physical and chemical filters. The chemical filters may lead to sensitization and then allergic (or photoallergic) contact dermatitis. In addition they can be irritating. For these reasons most experts recommend using physical blocking creams in children. They contain agents such as zinc oxide or titanium dioxide in elegant vehicles. One should also recommend a protective lip balm, as the lower lip is a major site of solar damage.

The sun, water and wind dry the skin out. Thus, after a day in the sun, an emollient cream should be applied to the skin. This step is especially important in children with dry skin or atopic dermatitis.

There may be medical reasons to avoid the sun. Children taking medications which lead to phototoxic or photoallergic reactions need to be warned. Two common acne medications, topical retinoids and tetracyclines, are phototoxic, meaning that the patients may have a lower threshold for a sunburn. Such individuals should be warned so they can adjust their exposure and protective habits accordingly. Furthermore, UV irradiation is somewhat immunosuppressive. Thus, children with a viral infection should probably avoid the sun for a few days. Herpes labialis may be triggered by sunlight and adequate sun protection is indicated to avoid recurrences of UV-induced herpes labialis.

References

Baker G. E., Driscoll M. S., Wagner R. F.: Emergency department management of sunburn reactions. Cutis 61:209–211 (1998)

Geller A. C., Coldlitz G., Oliveria S., Emmons K., Jorgensen C., Aweh G. N., Frazier A. L.: Use of sunscreen, sunburning rates, and tanning bed use among more than 10,000 US children and adolescents. Pediatrics 109:1009–1014 (2002)

Hurwitz S.: Clinical Pediatric Dermatology. Photosensitivity and Photoreactions, 2nd ed. W.B. Saunders, Philadelphia (1993)

Nguyen N. L., Gun R. T., Sparnon A. L., Ryan P.: The importance of immediate cooling – a case series of childhood burns in Vietnam. Burns 28:173–176 (2002)

Noonan F. P., Recio J. A., Takayama H., Duray P., Anver M. R., Rush W. L., De Fabo E. C., Merlino G.: Neonatal sunburn and melanoma in mice. Nature 413:2271–2272 (2001)

Palmieri T. L., Greenhalgh D. G.: Topical treatment of pediatric patients with burns: a practical guide. Am J Clin Dermatol 3:529–534 (2002)

CHAPTER 6 Diaper Dermatitis

K. Strom

Epidemiology

Diaper dermatitis is an extremely common skin disorder in infants and small children. At least 50% of children experience the problem at least once. The incidence is highest between 9 and 12 months of age.

Pathogenesis

Diaper dermatitis is triggered and worsened by a combination of physical, irritant, enzymatic and microbial factors. Occlusion by the diaper is the prime requirement. The occluded stratum corneum becomes more hydrated and is no longer as resistant to friction. The result is maceration which then favors colonization with *Candida albicans* and Gram-positive bacteria, especially *Staphylococcus aureus*. Bacteria with ureases are capable of splitting the uric acid in the urine producing ammonia which increases the pH value. In addition, the many enzymes present in stool add an additional irritating and inflammatory effect, some of them being activated by increased pH.

Clinical Features

The changes are not surprisingly limited to the diaper area. The initial finding is usually a glistening erythema (Fig. 15). As the disease progresses, erythematous macules and papules appear on an edematous background. Spreading outside the area of the diaper with collarette scale and pustules are often signs of candidal superinfection (Fig. 16). When in doubt, assume that a secondary candidal infection is present, as the likelihood is high in any diaper dermatitis persisting for more than 3 days. Finally erosions and even ulcers may develop; in Eu-

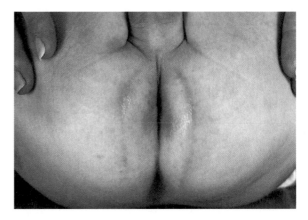

Fig. 15. Diaper dermatitis. Sharply localized perianal erythema.

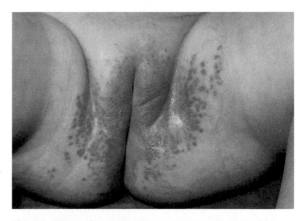

Fig. 16. Diaper dermatitis. More extensive disease with succulent papules, in some areas confluent, with typical satellite lesions suggesting associated *Candida albicans* infection.

rope this advanced stage is often designated Jacquet dermatitis.

Symptoms

The infants often scratch, suggesting that diaper dermatitis is quite pruritic.

Diagnosis

The diagnosis is clinical. Weeping or macerated areas should be cultured for *Candida albicans* and bacteria.

Differential Diagnosis

The major differential diagnostic considerations are shown in Table 18. The difference between intertrigo and diaper dermatitis is not well established. Intertrigo is a skin reaction that occurs when two skin surfaces come in contact, such as under the breasts or in the inguinal fold. In diaper dermatitis, often the skin folds where no diaper comes in contact with the skin are relatively spared. Thus, both processes involve moisture, rubbing, and maceration but are theoretically different. Clinically, they run together. In the

Table 18. Differential diagnosis of diaper dermatitis

Diagnosis	Distinguishing Features
■ **Intertrigo**	Irritation in skin folds where two surfaces rub against each other
■ **Atopic dermatitis**	Skin alterations not limited to diaper area; face and trunk usually involved; positive family history
■ **Seborrheic dermatitis**	Usually appears in first 12 weeks of life; other body areas involved, especially scalp and face
■ **Psoriasis**	Rarely limited to diaper area; usually involves scalp and face; often a positive family history
■ **Perianal streptococcal dermatitis**	Perianal infection with β-hemolytic streptococci; sharply localized; often painful

case of both *Candida albicans* and impetigo, the disease may also develop in the absence of diaper dermatitis. Extremely acute diaper dermatitis may be the presenting complaint of chickenpox starting out in an area of weakened skin. In the case of therapy-resistant diaper dermatitis, one should think of underlying diseases such as allergic contact dermatitis, psoriasis inversa, scabies, Langerhans cell histiocytosis and sexual abuse.

Therapy

■ **General Measures.** The bottom line is good nursing care. The diapers should be changed as soon as possible after the child has urinated or had a bowel movement. They should be changed at least once during the night. Extensive research and clinical experience has shown that super absorbent diapers are better than cotton diapers or other possibilities. Whenever feasible, the child should be let free to play or rest for a short time without diapers, if the parents are willing to risk an accident. Additional protective rubber or plastic underwear should be avoided. The diapers themselves are occlusive enough.

The second important measure in cleansing. Every mother and grandmother has their favorite approach. We recommend cleaning after each bowel movement with a mild synthetic detergent and water, or using a 1% clioquinol in zinc oil mixture.

■ Rx_
Clioquinol	1.0
Zinc oxide	50.0
Ol. oliv. ad	100.0

One can also influence the nature of the stool and urine through dietary measures. Infants who nurse have less diaper dermatitis, have a lower stool pH, and lower measurable enzyme activity. Cranberry juice (120–160 mL; 4–6 oz. daily) will lower the urine pH.

■ **Initial Treatment.** The basic principle of treating diaper dermatitis is to protect the skin from moisture and irritants and allow

Table 19. Therapy of diaper dermatitis

■ **Preventive measures**	Frequent change of diapers Cleansing after each bowel movement
■ **Standard therapy**	Protective pastes Astringent compresses
■ **Anti-inflammatory therapy**	Low-potency corticosteroids creams or ointments
■ **Antimicrobial therapy**	0.1% aqueous gentian violet solution; 1.0% chlorhexidine cream
■ **Anticandidal therapy**	Imidazole pastes or creams; rarely oral nystatin suspension
■ **Antibiotic therapy**	Fusidic acid products; systemic anti-staphylococcal agents

the skin to regenerate its natural barrier. If the diaper dermatitis is not weeping, then a purely protective paste such as zinc oxide paste can be used or absorbent pastes of the oil-in-water or water-in-oil type.

Two such pastes which we like to prescribe are:

W/O absorbent paste

■ Rx_
Zinc oxide	25.0
Wheat starch	25.0
Softisan 649	10.0
White vaseline ad	100.0

O/W absorbent paste

■ Rx_
Zinc oxide	25.0
Wheat starch	25.0
O/W ointment base ad	100.0

Cream paste

■ Rx_
Almond oil	20.0
Zinc oxide	20.0
Emollient cream base ad	100.0

When the diaper dermatitis is eroded, our first choice is 0.1% gentian violet in an aqueous solution painted on once daily. More frequent application and higher concentrations can, in rare cases, lead to necro-sis. Moist compresses soaked in an astringent solution such as black tea or synthetic tannic acid solutions can be applied for 30 minutes 2–3 times daily.

Other possibilities include an antiseptic paste or an anticandidal paste, commercially available in Germany as Imazol® paste.

Antiseptic paste

■ Rx_
Chlorhexidine gluconate	1.0
Zinc oxide	20.0
DAC Basis cream ad	50.0

■ **Anti-inflammatory Therapy.** Often good nursing care combined with astringent and protective measures is all that is required. In therapy-resistant cases, a low-potency corticosteroid cream, usually hydrocortisone but occasionally slighter stronger products or one of the new non-steroidal immunosuppressants (pimecrolimus, tacrolimus) can be applied 1–2 times daily for several days. Potent corticosteroids should be avoided, as under an occlusive diaper, systemic absorption and local side effects are both likely.

■ **Antimicrobial Therapy.** Gentian violet is a non-irritating astringent with a strong antimicrobial effect. Another possibility is chlorhexidine gluconate which can be added to creams or pastes in a 1% concentration.

When candidiasis is suspected, any of the imidazole derivatives are useful topically, such as clotrimazole, econazole or ketoconazole, best applied in the form of a cream paste. Combination products containing both an azole and a low-potency corticosteroid are helpful for 2–3 days. One should avoid the products such as triamcinolone acetonide-nystatin cream (Mycolog II®) or betamethasone dipropionate-clotrimazole (Lotrisone®) as the corticosteroid component is too high in potency for use in the diaper area.

Only rarely is systemic anticandidal therapy needed. The indications are a severe diaper dermatitis combined with oral candidiasis or repeatedly highly positive stool cultures for

Diaper Dermatitis

Candida albicans. The standard treatment is nystatin suspension 2 mL (200,000 IU) q.i.d. for 7 days.

If a staphylococcal impetigo is present, fusidic acid is the best agent. In Europe it comes as a cream, ointment, gel or powder. The imidazoles are also effective antibacterial agents, especially against Gram-positive bacteria, so they can be used when a mixed infection is suspected.

If a staphylococcal pustulosis or a clinically apparent impetigo develops (as contrasted to a positive skin culture), then systemic antibiotics are better. Either penicillinase-resistant penicillins or first-generation oral cephalosporins can be used. Erythromycin should only be chosen if the bacteria has been shown to be sensitive. In the case of penicillin allergy, clindamycin is the usual alternative.

References

Atherton D.J.: The aetiology and management of irritant diaper dermatitis. J Eur Acad Dermatol Venereol 15 (Suppl 1):1–4 (2001)

Berg R.W.: Etiology and pathophysiology of diaper dermatitis. Advances in Dermatology 3:75–98 (1988)

Concannon P., Gisoldi E., Phillips S., Grossman R.: Diaper dermatitis: a therapeutic dilemma. Results of a double-blind placebo controlled trial of miconazole nitrate 0.25%. Pediatr Dermatol 18:149–155 (2001)

Gloor M., Wolnicki D.: Anti-irritative effect to methylrosaniline chloride (gentian violet). Dermatology 203:325–328 (2001)

Jordan W.E., Lawson K.D., Berg R.W., Franxman J.J., Marrer A.M.: Diaper dermatitis: frequency and severity among general infant population. Pediatric Dermatology 3:198–207 (1986)

Wahrmann J.E., Honig P.J.: The management of diaper dermatitis – rational treatment based on specific etiology. Dermatological Therapy 2:9–17 (1997)

Weston W.L., Lane A.T., Weston J.A.: Diaper dermatitis: current concepts. Pediatrics 66:532–536 (1980)

CHAPTER 7

Granuloma Annulare

I. FORER

Epidemiology

Granuloma annulare is a common idiopathic benign granulomatous dermatosis which has a worldwide distribution. It is a generally asymptomatic, self-limited disease which is most common in the first three decades and affects twice as many women as men. Its incidence has been estimated at 0.1–0.4% of dermatologic patients.

Pathogenesis

The cause of granuloma annulare is unknown. In adults, there is some evidence of a link with diabetes mellitus, but this association has not even been suggested in children. Trauma may play a triggering role in localized and subcutaneous granuloma annulare, especially when the extremities are involved. Scattered case reports describe an association between granuloma annulare and both tuberculin skin testing and BCG immunization. On occasion, a relationship to autoimmune thyroiditis has been found.

The histological picture of granuloma annulare may also offer clues to its etiology. There is a central focus of necrobiotic (damaged) collagen surrounded by a lymphohistiocytic infiltrate arranged often in a palisade fashion – hence the term palisading granuloma, a feature also seen in rheumatoid nodules. The inflammatory cells are activated Th1 cells with the appropriate cytokine pattern, suggesting a T cell mediated immune response against specific (but unidentified) antigens. In addition, direct immunofluorescent examination reveals deposits of IgG and C3 around the dermal blood vessels, pointing to a possible immune complex vasculitis. Granuloma annulare may also develop in tattoos and in the scars associated with warts and herpes zoster, presumably as a non-specific immunologic reaction.

Clinical Features

Granuloma annulare is usually divided into localized, perforating, subcutaneous and disseminated variants.

■ **Localized Granuloma Annulare.** In children, over 90% of cases are the localized form. Typically a single or limited number of lesions are found on the extensor surfaces of the extremities (60% on the hands and arms, 20% on the feet and legs). In children, rare cases are found with periorbital involvement. Skin-colored or slightly erythematous firm dermal papules appear, usually arranged in an annular or arciform pattern with an unaffected central region (Figs. 17). The lesions may spread peripherally, partially resolve or recur at the same site. The epidermis is not involved.

■ **Subcutaneous Granuloma Annulare.** This form is found almost exclusively in children less than six years of age as solitary or multiple, clinically indistinct, deep dermal or subcutaneous nodules on the shin, forearm, elbow, back of the hand, fingers or especially the scalp. Once again the periorbital region,

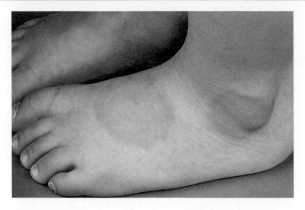

Fig. 17. Granuloma annulare. Annular lesion on dorsum of foot with typical subtle livid to red-brown color. The resemblance to "ring worm" (tinea corporis) is striking, but scales are not seen.

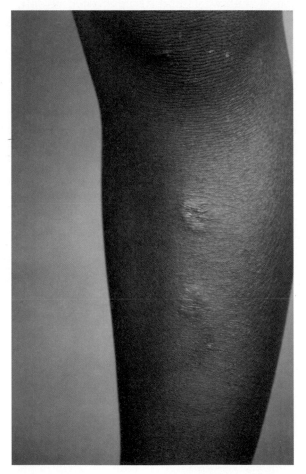

Fig. 18. Granuloma annulare. Disseminated form with less typical lesions.

usually the upper lid, may be affected. The nodules on the extremities are usually freely mobile although they may be attached to the fascia. In contrast, on the scalp, they are usually firmly fixed to the periosteum. In 25% of cases, more typical superficial lesions are also present. Even though the lesions are clinically and histologically similar to rheumatoid nodules, there is no connection between subcutaneous granuloma annulare and childhood rheumatoid arthritis.

■ **Perforating Granuloma Annulare.** About 5% of patients develop the perforating form of granuloma annulare. This is usually found on the hands or fingers and may simply be a traumatized variant of localized granuloma annulare. At least 50% of these patients are children or young adults. The papules develop central plugs, discharge a gelatinous material and then form crusts and umbilicated lesions. Later atrophic hypo- or hyperpigmented scars may develop. In the rare cases of disseminated perforating granuloma annulare, the typical clinical picture is that of papules which evolve into larger plaques. Perforating granuloma annulare is one of the prototypes of a perforating dermatosis, in which abnormal dermal tissue is discharged through the epidermis.

■ **Disseminated Granuloma Annulare.** This form is seen in about 15% of patients with granuloma annulare but is rare in children. The overwhelming majority of patients are more than 50 years of age. Skin-colored to violaceous grouped papules can be seen anywhere on the body, although the distal extremities and trunk are the most common sites (Fig. 18).

Symptoms

The lesions are almost always asymptomatic. Perforating granuloma annulare may be pruritic or painful.

Diagnosis

Granuloma annulare can usually be diagnosed clinically. Histological confirmation is often needed for subcutaneous granuloma annulare. Such cases can also be studied with magnetic resonance imaging, as the imaging picture can be easily recognized and more serious subcutaneous masses excluded.

Differential Diagnosis

The differential diagnostic considerations are shown in Table 20.

Therapy

The tendency of granuloma annulare to resolve spontaneously should be considered when planning therapy. About 75% of the lesions show spontaneous remission over a two year period. Although the recurrence rate is about 40%, the new lesions are also likely to disappear on their own. In addition, the process is asymptomatic and entirely benign, so following discussion with the parents, watchful waiting is often the best option.

If lesions are painful or disturb the patient, one can employ mid- to high-potency topical corticosteroids such as mometasone furoate each evening for 14 days, then every other evening for another 2–3 weeks. If mechanically possible, the lesions should be occluded. While topical vitamin E therapy has been endorsed, it is not effective in our hands. As occasionally a biopsy may lead to spontaneous resolution of a lesion, some individuals practice superficial scarification as a manner of treatment.

While a variety of systemic therapeutic options are available, none are clearly established as effective and none are recommended for pediatric patients. Included in the list are corticosteroids, dapsone, antimalarial drugs and retinoids, as well as PUVA and UVA1 phototherapy.

Table 20. 🍎 Diagnostic considerations

Diagnosis	Distinguishing Features
Localized granuloma annulare	
■ Tinea corporis	No papules; epidermal involvement with scaling; positive KOH and culture
■ Erythema elevatum diutinum	Not annular; deep red color; histologically a leukocytoclastic vasculitis
■ Erythema annulare centrifugum	Urticarial annular lesions; no papules; more rapidly peripheral spread; usually on trunk
Perforating granuloma annulare	
■ Elastosis perforans serpiginosa	Usually on nape; often associated with Down syndrome
Subcutaneous granuloma annulare	
■ Pilomatricoma	Usually on cheek; discharge of chalky material
■ Rheumatoid nodule	CAVEAT! Rheumatoid nodules rare in children; do not diagnose rheumatoid arthritis in asymptomatic child with necrobiotic nodule – it is granuloma annulare!
■ Foreign body granuloma	History; histological examination
■ Erythema nodosum	Usually on shin; appear as dusky red nodules resembling a bruise; associated with acute infections in some instances; painful to touch
Disseminated granuloma annulare	
■ Lichen planus	Violaceous flat topped papules; pruritus; often mucosal involvement

References

Cronquist S. D., Stashower M. E., Benson P. M.: Deep dermal granuloma annulare presenting as an eyelid tumor in a child, with review of pediatric eyelid lesions. Pediatric Dermatology 16:377–380 (1999)

Chung S., Frush D. P., Prose N. S., Shea C. R., Laor T., Bisset G. S.: Subcutaneous granuloma annulare: MR imaging features in six children and literature review. Radiology 210:845–8499 (1999)

Fond L., Michel J. L., Gentil-Perret A., Montelimard N., Perrot J. L., Chalencon V., Cambazard F.: Granulome annulaire de l'enfant. Arch Pédiatr 6:1017–1021 (1999)

Gradwell E., Evans S.: Perforating granuloma annulare complicating tattoos. Br J Dermatol 138:360–361(1998)

Grogg K. L., Nascimento A. G.: Subcutaneous granuloma annulare in childhood: clinicopathological features in 34 cases. Pediatrics 107:E42 (2001)

Houcke-Bruge C., Delaporte E., Catteau B., Martin De Lassalle E., Piette F.: Granuloma annulare following BCG vaccination. Ann Dermatol Venereol 128:541–544 (2001)

Jackson M. D., Pratt L., Lawson P.: Asymptomatic papules on a child. Perforating granuloma annulare. Arch Dermatol 137:1647–1652 (2001)

Kakurai M., Kiyosawa T., Ohtsuki M., Nakagawa H.: Multiple lesions of granuloma annulare following BCG vaccination: case report and review of the literature. Int J Dermatol 40:579–581 (2001)

Moran J., Lamb J.: Localized granuloma annulare and autoimmune thyroid disease. Are they associated? Can Fam Physician 41:2143–144 (1995)

Muhlemann M. F., Williams D. R. R.: Localized granuloma annulare is associated with insulin-dependent diabetes mellitus. Br J Dermatol 111:325–329 (1984)

Nebesio C. L., Lewis C., Chuang T. Y.: Lack of an association between granuloma annulare and type 2 diabetes mellitus. Br J Dermatol 146:122–124 (2002)

Salomon N., Walchner M., Messer G., Plewig G., Roecken M.: Bath-PUVA therapy of granuloma annulare. Hautarzt 50: 275–279 (1999)

Sandwich J. T., Davis L. S.: Granuloma annulare of the eyelid: a case report and review of the literature. Pediatric Dermatology 16:373–376 (1999)

Vazquez-Lopez F., Gonzalez-Lopez M. A., Raya-Aguado C., Perez-Oliva N.: Localized granuloma annulare and autoimmune thyroiditis: a new case report. J Am Acad Dermatol 43:943–945 (2000)

CHAPTER 8 Herpes Simplex Virus Infections

A. HEIDELBERGER

Epidemiology

The two herpes simplex viruses (HSV-1, HSV-2) belong to the group of human herpes viruses. Following the primary infection, they remain latent in for body for long periods of time, usually in neural tissue, only to become active again following a variety of triggers, causing secondary infections. An epidemiological survey in the US showed that 51% of persons aged 12 years and older were seropositive for HSV-1; 5.3% for HSV-2 and 16.6% both for HSV-1 and HSV-2, leaving only 27.1% negative for both.

HSV-1 typically involves the oropharynx and upper part of the body. The primary infection is known as herpetic gingivostomatitis and occurs in infants and toddlers as an acute febrile illness with extensive involvement of the oral mucosa. The secondary infection, herpes labialis, may be seen in older children and adolescents, usually localized without major systemic findings.

HSV-2 is more common on the genitalia and is of special interest to pediatricians because it can be spread during pregnancy and delivery leading to neonatal HSV infections with meningitis and sepsis. HSV-2 is generally acquired by sexual transmission. Primary infection in women (herpetic vulvovaginitis) can present as an acute, febrile, very painful illness with edema, blistering and erosions, but asymptomatic primary infection is also possible. The recurrences present during adult life as genital herpes simplex.

Pathogenesis

Both HSV-1 and HSV-2 are epidermotropic viruses. They are transferred by direct inoculation of skin or mucosal surfaces. The viruses multiply in the epithelial cells, and then may either spread via the blood or establish residence in the regional nerve ganglia.

Herpetic Gingivostomatitis

■ Clinical Features

The usual manner of infection is direct contact or droplet (kissing, sharing eating utensils or pacifiers). The initial sign is inflammation of the oral mucosa, soon followed by rapidly spreading blisters of varying sizes on the tongue, gingivae, palate, buccal mucosa and labial mucosa. The blisters ulcerate and become macerated producing typical 2 to 4 mm flat ulcers with a pseudomembrane (Fig. 19). The blisters and ulcers also extend to the perioral skin. The incubation period is 3 to 7 days and the period of infectivity may be several weeks.

Symptoms

The ulcers are painful and interfere with feeding. In addition, there may be increased salivation, an unpleasant mouth odor (known in German as *Mundfäule* = mouth rot), lymphadenopathy, fever, and irritability.

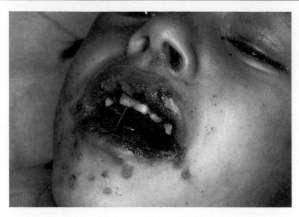

Fig. 19. Herpetic gingivostomatitis. Erosions of the lips and oral mucosa, some with hemorrhagic crusts, others with a necrotic membrane. Several perioral blisters, as well as nasal erosions.

Table 21. Differential diagnosis of herpetic gingivostomatitis

Diagnosis	Distinguishing Features
■ **Herpangina**	Caused by Coxsackie-A viruses; high fever (40 °C); tiny blisters on palate and tonsils with fibrin membrane and peripheral erythema; rarely large ulcers which resemble HSV
■ **Varicella**	Small ulcers with erythematous border in posterior oral cavity; characteristic lesions on scalp and trunk
■ **Infectious mononucleosis**	Usually oral petechiae, but occasionally gingivitis and jagged ulcers; lymphadenopathy and fever
■ **Plaut-Vincent gingivostomatitis**	Mixed bacterial infection in older children; usually poor oral hygiene
■ **Aphthae**	Usually 1 to 5 small ulcers with gray membrane and peripheral erythema; rarely on fixed mucosa

Diagnosis

The diagnosis is usually made clinically. Identification and typing of the virus are usually not needed. In confusing cases, direct immunofluorescent examination of blister fluid or scrapings from the base of an ulcer using monoclonal antibodies against type specific viral capsule glycoproteins gives the quickest and most reliable diagnostic confirmation.

Differential Diagnosis

If there are not perioral findings, the diagnosis may be almost overlooked, as the parents blame the child's difficulty in feeding to teething or changes in diet. The differential diagnostic considerations are shown in Table 21.

Therapy

■ Acyclovir

Oral antiviral therapy should be instituted, usually using an acyclovir suspension. The recommended dosage is 15 mg/kg daily in 5 divided doses for 7 days. If the child is un-

able to take the oral medication, then hospitalization with intravenous administration may be required.

■ **Supportive Measures.** Careful gentle oral hygiene is important. We have found it useful to use a "numbing" mouthwash prior to eating and a "cleansing" wash afterwards (Table 22). Products contain benzocaine should be avoided as it is such a potent contact allergen. Fluid and electrolyte replacement as well as control of fever are the other important measures, especially in infants. Once again, sometimes hospitalization is needed to accomplish this task.

Complications

The main complication is difficulty in eating and drinking, leading to dehydration. Secondary bacterial infections, most often impetigo may occur. Sometimes the lymphadenopathy evolves into lymphadenitis. Often the child also develops lesions on the hands, especially their thumbs, as a result of viral transmission during thumb sucking.

Table 22. Treatment of herpetic gingivostomatitis

Systemic therapy	Acyclovir suspension 15 mg/kg daily divided in 5 doses
Topical therapy*	
Numbing	
■ Dynexan A® Gel	1 g of gel contains 20 mg of lidocaine and 1 mg of benzalkonium chloride; a pea-sized piece can be massaged into the gums before eating
■ Herviros® Solution	100 g contain 0,5 g aminoquinuride hydrochloride, 1 g tetracaine hydrochloride; apply with cotton-tipped applicator before meals
Cleansing	
■ Hexetidin solution	rinse or clean with cotton-tipped applicator after meals and as desired
■ Chamomile tea solution	as above

* We recognize many of these products are only available in Germany but the physician can substitute local equivalents.

Herpes Simplex Labialls

■ Clinical Features

The typical finding here is grouped vesicles and blisters on an erythematous base, usually on the skin immediately adjacent to the lips (Fig. 20). Such lesions are known to everyone as fever blisters or cold sores, because the trigger is so often a viral or bacterial infection with fever. Another common trigger is sunlight. The blisters rupture, dry out and develop a brown crust. Cloudy blister fluid or thick yellowish crusts may be a sign of bacterial secondary infection. The lesions usually heal without scarring.

A common complication is the development of erythema multiforme. Patients with blisters or draining lesions are infectious and should avoid contact with newborn infants and immunosuppressed individuals. When contact cannot be avoided, a mask should be worn.

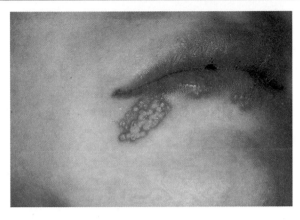

Fig. 20. Herpes simplex labialis. Multiple grouped (herpetiform) blisters, most filled with pus, on an erythematous background.

Symptoms

In most cases, the patient experiences an abnormal sensation hours before the erythema or blisters appear. Some may describe pain; others, burning, but almost everyone senses something. The active lesions may also be painful.

Diagnosis

The diagnosis can almost always be made clinically.

Differential Diagnosis

Almost all perioral recurrent lesions are HSV. In rare cases, most uncommonly in children, one cannot distinguish with certain between a large unilateral lesion of HSV and a small lesion of herpes zoster. In such cases, virological studies should be performed.

Similarly, it can be difficult to distinguish between a secondarily infected herpes labialis and impetigo. The patient should be asked to present to a physician as soon as possible should the lesion recur, so that the early signs of HSV can be sought.

Therapy

Specific antiviral therapy is usually not necessary and does not markedly influence the severity or duration of the illness. Topical acyclovir therapy is not effective. In patients who have frequent recurrences or associated erythema multiforme, prophylactic therapy with systemic acyclovir should be considered. We usually prescribe acyclovir for 6 or 12 months in the range of 5 mg/kg daily in two divided dosages. Dose adjustment may be needed to maintain suppression.

Topical drying and antiseptic measures are very helpful. We prefer a zinc oxide shake lotion with 1% chlorhexidine gluconate or a tannic acid shake lotion. If secondary impetiginization has occurred, we usually use fusidic acid ointment 3 or 4 times daily. An active immunization to prevent recurrent herpes simplex infections is not yet available, but several vaccines are currently undergoing testing.

■ Other Types of HSV-1 Infections

■ Recurrent Herpes Simplex at Other Sites. One should suspect HSV secondary infection anytime a patient reports that a skin lesion reappears on the same spot. While the most typical site is perioral, HSV can recur at any site of inoculation (Fig. 21). In adults the most typical extra-oral, extra-genital site is the buttocks; in children, acral lesions are more common. When vesicles or pustules are present, the diagnosis is easier than if only crusts or erosions are seen, which is so often the case. Once again, the patient should be ask to present again as early as possible if the lesions recur.

■ Herpes Simplex Encephalitis. This is the most common form of viral encephalitis, almost always caused by HSV-1. About 1/3 of the patients are under 20 years of age. The fatality rate is 70–80%. Most patients do not have associated cutaneous disease. While early diagnosis is crucial, the signs and symptoms are

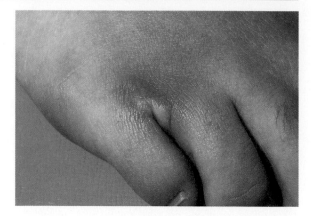

Fig. 21. Recurrent herpes simplex in the interdigital space, with a large pus-filled blister surrounded by erythema.

not specific, with either flu-like symptoms or headache. Magnetic resonance imaging is the preferred diagnostic approach and high-dose intravenous acyclovir should be instituted as rapidly as possible.

■ Eczema Herpeticatum. This devastating illness represents the widespread cutaneous dissemination of HSV in damaged or susceptible skin. Most victims have atopic dermatitis, although the same problem can be seen in burns, Darier disease, Hailey-Hailey disease and several other situations. Many patients are children, and HSV-1 is most often responsible.

The usual method of infection is exogenous, following contact with individuals who have herpes labialis and then a primary infection. In some cases, a secondary infection can spread causing endogenous eczema herpeticum. Key factors in the pathogenesis are the weakened barrier function of atopic skin and often the use of topical corticosteroids.

The clinical picture is one of severe systemic disease with fever and malaise, associated with multiple small vesicles which later become confluent, eroded, often hemorrhagic and are easily secondarily infected. The skin changes can remain localized to the areas of dermatitis (localized eczema herpeticum) or spread to involve normal skin (generalized eczema herpeticum). The most likely sites of involvement are the face, neck and arms.

Systemic antiviral therapy is required. Usually acyclovir 5–10 mg/kg t.i.d. for 7 days is sufficient. It should be started as soon as possible. If all of the lesions are dry and crusted, the acyclovir is no longer helpful. In addition, topical antiseptic (triclosan 1–2% cream) or antibiotic (fusidic acid ointment) agents are useful. If the bacterial secondary infection is severe, oral antibiotics may also be appropriate. Usually either a first generation oral cephalosporin or penicillinase-resistant penicillin is chosen.

■ **Herpetic Keratoconjunctivitis.** Involvement of the cornea can lead to erosions, which are painful and may cause scarring and reduce vision. Over 60% of patients develop astigmatism. If herpetic ocular disease is suspected, the patient should be referred immediately to an ophthalmologist for emergency consultation.

■ **Post-herpetic Erythema Multiforme.** One of the common complications of herpes labialis is erythema multiforme, which typically develops 1 to 2 weeks after the viral infection. The usual site of involvement is the dorsal aspects of the hands where iris or target lesions develop. Individual lesions have three zones: central hemorrhage, a surrounding cyanotic zone and then peripheral bright erythema. Sometimes the lesions can be more widespread, but this is more common in drug-related erythema multiforme. Mucosal involvement occurs and can be difficult to distinguish from the triggering herpetic lesion.

Treatment is based on the severity of the disease. If only a few relatively asymptomatic lesions are present, no treatment is needed. If the lesions are pruritic, mid-potency topical corticosteroids can be tried. Widespread disease as well as mucosal involvement may indicate the need for systemic corticosteroids; we usually use methylprednisolone 1 mg/kg daily for 3 days and then taper rapidly. The theoretical risk of dissemination of the HSV during corticosteroid therapy is fortunately not a clinical problem. Patients with recurrent post-herpetic erythema multiforme are good candidates for acyclovir prophylaxis as discussed above.

References

Amir J., Harel L., Smetana Z., Varsana I.: Treatment of herpes simplex gingivostomatitis with aciclovir in children: a randomised double blind placebo controlled study. British Medical Journal 314:1800–1803 (1997)

Beigi B., Algawi K., Foley-Nolan A., O'Kufe M.: Herpes simplex keratitis in children. British Journal of Ophthalmology 78:458–460 (1994)

Forman R., Koren G., Shear N.H.: Erythema multiforme, Stevens-Johnson syndrome and toxic epidermal necrolysis in children: a review of 10 years' experience. Drug Saf 25:965–972 (2002)

Nathwani D., Wood M.J.: Herpes infections in childhood. British Journal of Hospital Medicine 50:233–241 (1993)

Nikkels A.F., Perard G.E.: Treatment of mucocutaneous presentations of herpes simplex virus infections. Am J Clin Dermatol 3:475–487 (2002)

Stanberry L.R., Rosenthal S.L.: Genital herpes simplex virus infection in the adolescent: special considerations for management. Paediatr Drugs 4:291–297 (2002)

Walker L.G., Simmons B.P., Lovallo J.L.: Pediatric herpetic hand infections. Journal of Hand Surgery 15:176–179 (1990)

Xu F., Schillinger J.A., Sternberg M.R., Johnson R.E., Lee F.K., Nahmias A.J., Markowitz L.E.: Seroprevalence and coinfection with herpes simplex virus type 1 and type 2 in the United States, 1988–1994. J Infect Dis 185:1019–1024 (2002)

CHAPTER 9 Impetigo

M. MEMPEL

Epidemiology

Impetigo is a common contagious cutaneous infection which appears almost exclusively in childhood. Up to 10% of patients in a general pediatric outpatient clinic may have impetigo.

Pathogenesis

The causative organisms of impetigo are Gram-positive cocci, mainly *Staphylococcus aureus* and group A streptococci (*Streptococcus pyogenes*). Infections with *Staphylococcus aureus* are far more common. The traditional division into bullous impetigo from *Staphylococcus aureus* and non-bullous from *Streptococcus pyogenes* is incorrect. The skin is infected by invasion of the upper layers of the epidermis by the bacteria where especially the exfoliative toxins from *S. aureus* (ETA-ETD) cause blister formation by proteolytic digestion of the desmoglein 1 showing parallels to pemphigus foliaceus. This process is facilitated by microtrauma to the skin such as scratches. The dramatic inflammatory events are mediated by proinflammatory enzymes which the bacteria release such as proteases, lipases, nucleases and others.

Clinical Features

The initial lesion of impetigo consists of vesicles and blisters on an erythematous background. Sometimes the blisters are tense; in other instances, they are flaccid. In either event, they rupture easily and rapidly, and there is massive exudation of tissue fluid forming characteristic honey-colored to brown thick crusts with peripheral erythema (Fig. 22). In German, these crusts are called *Borken*, referring to the bark of a tree. The corner of the mouth is often affected, producing angular cheilitis (perlèche). Sometimes widespread areas are involved (Fig. 23). The lesions usually heal without scarring. Regional lymphadenopathy may develop.

Symptoms

Some patients are relatively asymptomatic while others are quite ill with malaise and fever.

Diagnosis

While the diagnosis is usually clinically straight-forward, it should be confirmed by microbiological methods. While therapy should be started based on the clinical diagnosis alone, the culture and sensitivity results are useful in the event of a failure to respond to treatment or the appearance of complications. In addition, we monitor the urine at the time of diagnosis and two weeks after treatment is concluded.

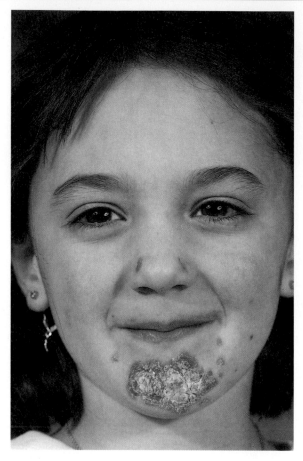

Fig. 22. Impetigo. Honey-colored crusts on erythematous base on chin. Tiny satellite lesions also seen.

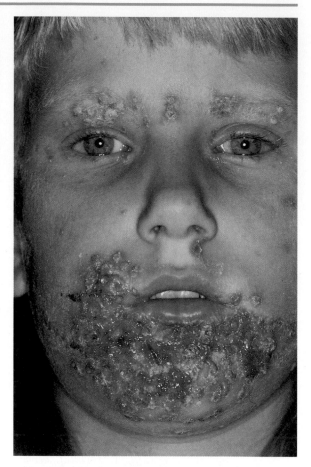

Fig. 23. Impetigo. More disseminated disease with massive involvement of chin and perioral region. Intact pustules, honey-colored crusts and hemorrhagic crusts are all seen.

Differential Diagnosis

In most cases the only question is – does the patient have impetigo or an impetiginized dermatitis? Other differential diagnostic considerations are shown in Table 23.

Therapy

The main issue is the relative roles of topical and systemic therapy. Localized lesions can usually be treated effectively with topical measures but widespread disease, appearance at multiple sites simultaneously and systemic signs and symptoms all suggest a need for systemic treatment. In general, pa-

Table 23. Differential diagnosis of impetigo

Diagnosis	Distinguishing Features
■ **Herpes simplex**	Grouped clear vesicles; often recurrent; usually burning or pain prior to appearance of lesions; frequently secondarily impetiginized
■ **Folliculitis**	Pustules involving hair follies; no honey-colored crusts and only rarely confluent lesions; usually caused by staphylococci
■ **Acne vulgaris**	Onset in puberty; pustules plus comedones

tients treated with systemic antibiotics heal somewhat faster and become non-infectious sooner, an important attribute for their siblings and classmates. Early systemic treatment may reduce the incidence of post-streptococcal glomerulonephritis and rheumatic fever through the prevention of an active immune response against streptococci.

■ **Topical Therapy.** The best topical antibiotic for staphylococci and streptococci in Europe is fusidic acid. It is available in a variety of vehicles (gel, cream, ointment), offering therapeutic flexibility. It is especially effective against staphylococci, including penicillinase-resistant strains. Mupirocin is similarly effective, but should be reserved for MRSA elimination in high-risk patients. Another alternative is gentamicin ointment. All should be applied t.i.d. for 7–10 days. It is wise to gently soak the thick crusts before each application, as once they are softened and removed, penetration is better.

We recommend not using neomycin products, as they are relatively ineffective, often lead to resistance, and may cause contact dermatitis. Topical tetracycline and erythromycin products are also not wise, as the resistance to these agents is quite high in most communities. Topical antiseptics are not as effective as antibiotics but can be used in conjunction with systemic measures.

■ **Systemic Therapy.** The definite choice of an antibiotic is usually based on the results of the bacterial culture and sensitivity. Initially one chooses an antibiotic effective against *Staphylococcus aureus* which also is effective against streptococci. The two recommended agents are first generation oral cephalosporins and the combination of amoxicillin and clavulanic acid (Table 24). The most common side effects of both of these agents are exanthems. In the case of penicillin allergy, clindamycin is a reasonable substitute. All are available in suspensions for pediatric use. The standard duration of therapy is 10 days.

Erythromycin has long been the preferred agent because of its lack of side effects, but the increasing resistance of staphylococci has restricted its use. Up to 30% of the strains of staphylococci have been shown be resistant to erythromycin in different studies worldwide. The same resistance problems exist with the newer macrolide antibiotics. This entire family should only be employed after sensitivity has been demonstrated.

■ **Recurrent Disease.** If a patient has recurrent impetigo, the first step is to administer systemic therapy if the previous infection was handled topically. The next approach is to identify nasal or less often perianal carriage, which is usually the reservoir for the staphylococci. One possible approach to eliminating the carrier status is to apply mupirocin ointment to the nares (not just the anterior nares [vestibule] but as far up as possible) b.i.d. for 1 week and then once a week for a long period of time. Protocols involving clindamycin or rifampicin are also available in the literature, but expert consultation should be sought at this point.

■ **Supportive Measures.** The skin should be washed with disinfectant synthetic detergents. In addition, an antiseptic cream (1% chlorhexidine gluconate or 2% triclosan in a cream base) can be used for routine skin care. Children should be kept away from kindergarten or school until they have ceased to develop new lesions.

■ **Complications.** There are a variety of complications. Streptococci may cause glomerulonephritis (reaction to M surface antigens), endocarditis (often *Streptococcus viridans*) and Sydenham chorea. The later are rarely seen in skin infections but one should keep in mind that transient colonization of the skin often proceeds to overt infections of the throat. Although the entire mechanism is not clear yet, it has been nicely shown that streptococci can aggravate psoriasis by the skin infiltration of cross-reacting T cell clones.

Staphylococci can cause soft tissue infections and osteomyelitis but these problems

Table 24. Systemic treatment of impetigo

Antibiotic	Form	Contents	Dose
■ **Cephalexin**	Tablet	500 mg, 1000 mg	≥14 y.: 1.5–3.0 g daily in 3 divided doses
	Liquid	50 mg/mL	0–14 y.: 25–100 mg/kg daily
■ **Amoxicillin and clavulanic acid**	Tablet	500 mg amox; 125 mg clav	>12 y., >40 kg: 1 tab t.i.d.
	Liquid	25 mg amox; 6.25 mg clav/mL	0–2 y.: 37.5 mg amox/kg daily in 3 divided doses 2–12 y.: 50 mg amox/kg daily in 3 divided doses
	Drops	50 mg amox; 12 mg clav/mL	<2 y.: 37.5 mg/kg in 3 divided doses
with penicillin allergy			
■ **Clindamycin**	Capsule	75–150–300 mg	>14 y.: 1200–1800 mg daily in 3–4 divided doses >4 weeks–14 y.: 8–25 mg/kg daily in 3–4 divided doses
	Liquid	15 mg/mL	>4 weeks–14 y.: 8–25 mg/kg daily in 3–4 divided doses

are limited almost entirely to immunosuppressed children. Some strains of staphylococci found in impetigo produce exfoliative toxins responsible for staphylococcal scalded skin syndrome; this possibility should be kept in mind in the case of rapidly spreading bullous disease in younger children. Patients should be monitored appropriately for all these complications.

References

Abeck D., Mempel M., Seidl H.P., Schnopp C., Ring J., Heeg K.: Impetigo contagiosa – Erregerspektrum und therapeutische Konsequenzen. Deutsche Medizinische Wochenschrift 125:1257–1259 (2000)

Abeck D., Korting H.C., Mempel M.: Pyodermien. Hautarzt 49:243–252 (1998)

Amagai M., Matsuyoshi N., Wang Z.H., Andl C., Stanley J.R.: Toxin in bullous impetigo and staphylococcal scalded-skin syndrome targets desmoglein 1. Nature Med 6:1275–1277 (2000)

Cunningham M.W.: Pathogenesis of group A streptococcal infections. Clin Microbiol Rev 13:470–511 (2000)

Darmstadt G.L., Lane A.T.: Impetigo: an overview. Pediatr Dermatol 11:293–303 (1994)

Epstein M.E., Amodio-Groton M., Sadick N.S.: Antimicrobial agents for the dermatologist. I. β-lactam antibiotics and related compounds. Journal of the American Academy of Dermatology 37:149–165 (1997)

Epstein M.E., Amodio-Groton M., Sadick N.S.: Antimicrobial agents for the dermatologist. II. Macrolides, fluoroquinolones, rifamycins, tetracyclines, trimethoprim-sulfamethoxazole, and clindamycin. Journal of the American Academy of Dermatology 37:365–381 (1997)

Koning S., van Suijlekom-Smit L.W.A., Nouwen J.L., Verduin C.M., Bernsen R.M.D, Oranje A.P., Thomas S., van der Wouden J.C.: Fusidic acid cream in the treatment of impetigo in general practice: double blind randomised placebo controlled trial. BMJ 324:1–5 (2002)

Prinz J.C.: Psoriasis vulgaris–a sterile antibacterial skin reaction mediated by cross-reactive T cells? An immunological view of the pathophysiology of psoriasis. Clin Exp Dermatol 6:326–332 (2001)

Simon C., Stille W.: Antibiotika-Therapie in Klinik und Praxis, 10. Auflage. Schattauer, Stuttgart, New York (2000)

Chapter 10   Lice Infestations

O. Brandt

Epidemiology

There are three different lice which may affect humans. Only one is a major problem in pediatrics. The head louse, *Pediculus humanus capitis*, can involve individuals of all ages and social strata. The prevalence is 1–3% in industrialized countries. Transmission is usually by direct head-to-head contact, which explains why most patients are children between 3 and 11 years of age. Shared combs, brushes, headgear and pillows can also lead to infestation. In contrast, pets do not play a role in the transmission of head lice. Hair length and hair color play no role. There are seasonal variations in the prevalence. In Europe, the winter months show the highest rates. Occasionally epidemics are seen in kindergartens and schools. The head louse does not transmit any infectious diseases.

In contrast the body louse, *Pediculus humanus humanus*, most typically involves individuals with inadequate hygiene. It is uncommon in western Europe but seen more often in the eastern regions. In the USA, the infestation is known as vagabond's skin. Homeless individuals, or those who are unable or unwilling to practice simple personal hygiene and launder their clothes, are at risk. Not surprisingly, body lice are often a problem among military units. Transmission is by personal contact, clothing or bedding. The body louse is the vector for a number of infectious diseases including epidemic typhus, trench fever, and relapsing fever.

The pubic louse, *Phthirus pubis*, is usually found first after puberty in pubic hairs. While it can be spread by sexual contact, transmission by fomites is also possible. Small children may acquire the infestation from adults, in which case it tends to involve the eyebrows and eyelashes.

Pathogenesis

Lice are wingless blood-sucking insects with three pairs of legs in the Suborder Anoplura. The lice simply transfer themselves from one individual or an inert object to their new host. The females have an accessory gland near the ovary which produces a water-insoluble glue which they use to attach their eggs (nits). All cause skin lesions by inserting their mouth parts, injecting saliva with toxic and proteolytic enzymes and then enjoying a blood meal.

The female head louse is 2–3.5 mm long and can be seen with the naked eye. During her reproductive life of 20–40 days, she lays 3–9 eggs daily which she attaches to hairs close to the skin surface. Head lice ingest a blood meal every 4–6 hours and can only live for 24 hours in the absence of a live host.

The adult body louse is slightly larger than the head louse, up to 4.5 mm, lays 5–14 eggs daily and has a life expectancy of 40 days. Body lice live on the clothing and only leave it for their meals. They lay their eggs in the seams of the clothing. They can survive much longer without a host, up to one week.

Pubic lice are smaller, about 1.7 mm, and have a squat body in contrast to the more elongated body of the head and body lice.

They are known as "crabs" for this reason. They are hard to see, but can be identified moving about the pubic hairs. Their nits are easier to find. Pubic lice live for about 30 days, producing 1–3 eggs daily. They can live up to three days in the absence of a host.

Clinical Features

Head lice favor the occipital and retroauricular regions of the scalp. Other hairy areas are seldom involved. Their nits are attached firmly like buds to the hair shafts and do not brush off, in contrast to dandruff scales (Fig. 24). At the sites of feeding, initially one sees only small petechial bleeding. A few hours later an intensely pruritic papule evolves. The combination of repeated scratching, chronic disease and a moist environment often leads to a dermatitis and secondary infection with *Staphylococcus aureus* or *Streptococcus pyogenes* (Fig. 25). Some children may have fever, lymphadenopathy, and other general signs of infection.

Body lice tend to bite in areas where the clothing restricts their movements, such as around the neck, shoulders, belt line and buttocks. The first lesions are typically urticarial papules or firm nodules, followed by excoriations, lichenification and superinfection involving large areas of the body. This is rarely seen in children in industrialized countries.

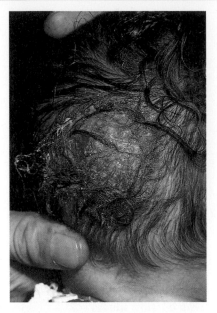

Fig. 25. Secondarily infected dermatitis associated with head lice infestation. Weeping erythema with yellow crusts, as well as occasional nits.

In the case of pubic lice, the bite sites tend to be more hemorrhagic and after 8–24 hours develop a distinctive blue-gray color. The irregular, several mm in diameter lesions are known as maculae ceruleae. Excoriations are uncommon. In small children, there may be extensive involvement of the eyelashes and eyebrows (phthiriasis palpebrarum). In extreme cases, the infestation can make it impossible to open the eyelids.

Symptoms

Infestations with head and body lice tend to be extremely pruritic; those with pubic lice much less so. Pruritus first becomes prominent after the host has been sensitized to the proteins in the louse saliva. This typically takes several weeks. If a re-infestation occurs, the pruritus develops in a matter of hours.

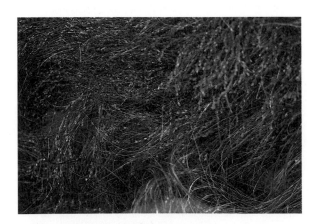

Fig. 24. Multiple nits of head lice.

Diagnosis

The gold standard of diagnosis is of course finding the bug. The diagnosis of head lice or pubic lice is confirmed by identifying the nits which are usually easier to find than the organisms. Using a nit comb may be a more sensitive and faster way to detect lice and nits than simple inspection. If only nits are present, the risk of conversion to active lice infestation is very small if they are found further than 6 mm from the scalp. If body lice are suspected, the clothing should be searched carefully.

Differential Diagnosis

In the case of pediculosis capitis, other inflammatory diseases of the scalp should be excluded, as shown in Table 25. The better approach is to be certain to exclude head lice before diagnosing impetigo or other scalp disorders.

Therapy

There are a wide variety of preparations available for treating lice infestations (Table 26). Medicated shampoos are less effective than products that are applied to the scalp and hairs for a longer period of time. In all instances, direct contact with the mucosal surfaces and eyes should be avoided. No matter what treatment is chosen, the patient should be carefully re-examined 7–10 days after conclusion of treatment, searching for lice and nits. Presence of multiple living lice 1–2 days after treatment suggest a treatment failure; a single louse is more likely to represent re-infestation. If treatment fails, improper use of medication is the likely explanation, but increasing levels of resistance of head lice against pyrethrins and permethrin are being reported from Central Europe and the United States. Thus, the use of another agent should be considered.

Table 25. Differential diagnosis of pediculosis capitis

Diagnosis	Distinguishing Features
■ **Atopic dermatitis**	Involvement of other typical sites; positive history; no nits
■ **Psoriasis**	Less pruritus; typical involvement of hairline; other evidence for psoriasis; no nits

Table 26. Treatment of lice infestations

Medication	Dosage	Duration
■ **Allethrin (spray)**	single use	30 minutes
■ **Permethrin (0.5%)**	two treatments, one week apart	30–45 minutes
■ **Lindane (gel 0.3%)**	two treatments, one week apart	3 days
■ **Pyrethrum extract**	two treatments, one week apart	30 minutes
■ **Malathion (0.5% lotion)**	two treatments, 8–10 days apart	8–12 hours

■ **Allethrin.** Sprays containing allethrin can be used against all three forms of lice. When treating head lice, one must be certain to treat the nape, temples and especially the scalp itself, not just to spray the hairs. The hairs can be washed after 30 minutes with any shampoo. The lice and nits must then be combed out with a fine-toothed comb.

■ **Permethrin.** The most reliable agent for the treatment of head and body lice is permethrin used in a concentration of 0.5%–1%. The solution is applied to the freshly washed scalp, allowed to work for 30–45 minutes and then rinsed out with warm water. The hairs should not be washed for three days. A single application cures over 90% of cases. Pubic lice should be re-treated after one week.

■ **Lindane (gamma benzene hexachloride).** Lindane is less effective in killing eggs than permethrin, so the treatment course should be repeated after one week. After washing the hair with an ordinary shampoo, the lindane gel is rubbed in the hairs and dispersed by repeated combing. It is removed by washing on the fourth day.

■ **Pyrethrum Extract.** One of the most popular products for eliminating lice available in Germany is Goldgeist forte®, a mixture of pyrethrum extracts. The liquid is rubbed into the involved areas, left on for 30 minutes and then rinsed out. No more than 25 mL should be used when treating infants and small children; it is recommended that infants be treated under medical observation. A second cycle of treatment should be performed 7–10 days later as pyrethrum does not kill nits.

■ **Malathion.** Malathion, an organophosphate, has been approved as a 0.5% lotion for head lice infestations. As it is effective against lice and nits, a single application is usually sufficient. Resistance is rare, so it is suitable as a second-line treatment. Malathion has neurotoxic side-effects and should therefore used with care in young children where absorption through the skin is greater.

■ **Eyelash and Eyebrow Involvement.** None of the above agents lend themselves to treating the periocular hairs. Ophthalmic ointments with sympathomimetic agents such as pilocarpine or neostigmine are the treatment of choice. They must be applied directly to the involved hairs and not allowed to come in contact with the eyes, because they cause mydriasis and myopia, leading to temporary visual impairment, especially for driving. Another approach is to use ordinary Vaseline to coat the nits and then remove them with a fine tweezers. We usually treat the scalp simultaneously with permethrin.

■ **Other Methods.** Heat is sometimes recommended as a treatment but it is clearly not as effective as a pharmaceutical approach. The patient must tolerate temperatures greater than 65 °C or more for at least 30 minutes. Sometimes saunas are employed to achieve these temperatures. Studies have shown that repeated combing (up to one hour daily) alone is not as effective as using medications.

■ **Removal of Nits.** Nits can be best removed by soaking the hairs with a solution of table vinegar (1 part): water (2 parts) for 30 minutes and then repeated combing with a nit comb. Mechanical removal of nits is important as medication penetrates poorly the nit shell.

■ **Supportive Measures.** Parents, siblings, and all others with close contact to a proven case should be inspected closely and treated if there are any suspicious findings. If pruritus is severe, systemic antihistamines can be given until the infestation is under control. We use doxylamine succinate, dimethindene maleate or hydroxyzine.

The inflamed, irritated skin should be treated twice daily with a basic non-medicated cream or lotion. If the irritation is marked, a low potency corticosteroid cream or lotion can be used for several days. Finally, bacterial secondary infections should treated with a penicillinase-resistant penicillin or a first generation cephalosporin.

Clothing (especially headgear!) and bedding should be washed at a temperature of at least 60 °C or commercially dry cleaned. If one wishes to avoid chemicals or has clothing which cannot be easily washed or cleaned, one can starve the lice. The materials must be isolated for at least one week. Alternatively, smaller items can be placed in a sealed plastic bag and then left in a freezer for 24–48 hours. Combs and brushes can be cleaned for 15 minutes in hot soapy water and can then safely be reused.

Finally, many girls have sacrificed long hair because of the mistaken belief that it was a predisposing factor for their head louse infestation. Hair length play no role in either acquiring or eliminating the infestation, except in the situation if one is trying to treat by combing alone, where shorter hairs are simpler to comb.

■ **Absence from School/Kindergarten.** Children should be kept away from school as long as they have live lice. Any of the above medical treatments kills such a high percentage of the lice that the risk of spread is very small following a single treatment. Thus, the children can return to school or kindergarten following the initial therapy. Rules prohibiting children with nits from returning are overcautious and not necessary.

References

Meinking T.L., Taplin D.: Infestations. In: Schachner L.A., Hansen R.C. (eds.) Pediatric Dermatology, 2nd ed., pp. 1347–1367. Churchill Livingstone, New York (1995)

Meinking T.L., Taplin D.: Infestations: Pediculosis. Current Problems in Dermatology 24:157–163 (1996)

Meinking T.L., Serrano L., Hard B., Entzel P., Lemard G., Rivera E., Villar M.E.: Comparative in vitro pediculocidal efficacy of treatments in a resistant head lice population in the United States. Arch Dermatol 138:220–224 (2002)

Molinari F.: Update on the treatment of pediculosis and scabies. Pediatric Nursing 18:600–602 (1992)

Roberts R.J.: Head lice. N Engl J Med 346:1645–1650 (2002)

Roberts R.J., Casey D., Morgan D.A., Petrovic M.: Comparison of wet combing with malathion for treatment of head lice in the UK: a pragmatic randomised controlled trial. Lancet 356:540–544 (2000)

Treating head lice. Atlanta: Centers for Disease Control. *http://www.cdc.gov/ncidod/dpd/parasites/headlice*

Williams L.K., Reichert A., MacKenzie W.R., Hightower A.W., Blake P.A.: Lice, nits, and school policy. Pediatrics 107:1011–1015 (2001)

Lice Infestations

CHAPTER 11

Lichen Sclerosus et Atrophicus

S. Thomsen

Epidemiology

Lichen sclerosus et atrophicus (LSA) shows a marked female predominance, up to 10:1 in some studies. Prevalence figures for childhood are not available, but in our experience the disease is clearly underdiagnosed.

Pathogenesis

The cause of LSA is unknown. The two most popular explanations are an autoimmune basis (HLA associations, diverse autoantibodies, overlaps with morphea, association with autoimmune disease, positive family history) and an infectious nature (in Europe, perhaps *Borrelia burgdorferi*).

Clinical Features

Anogenital LSA is much more common than extragenital disease. The extragenital disease is found in about 20% of cases, either isolated or in association with typical anogenital changes. Extragenital LSA is almost entirely restricted to girls.

The extragenital lesions are most common in pressure areas such as the nape or belt line, suggesting a possible Köbner response to trauma. The lesions are small white glistening papules with a cigarette paper-like wrinkling of the surface and prominent follicular ostia. As the disease progresses, 0.5–1.0 cm porcelain or blue-white, oval flat or atrophic patches develop. They often have peripheral erythema and may have follicular keratotic plugs (Fig. 26).

In the anogenital region, sharply defined white patches are seen with peripheral erythema and occasionally central hyperkeratotic areas. More severe cases display erosions, hemorrhage and even hemorrhagic blisters (Fig. 27). Bacterial and fungal secondary infections are occasionally seen and may be an aggravating factor. Infantile pyramidal protrusion refers to a bulging between the rectum and vagina along the perineal line which is also seen primarily in young girls, can also cause clinical confusion, and is histologically LSA.

In boys, the usual clinical finding is a scarring phimosis (Fig. 28) which is often not diagnosed as LSA. Often the histological examination of the circumcision specimen gives the first clue to the diagnosis.

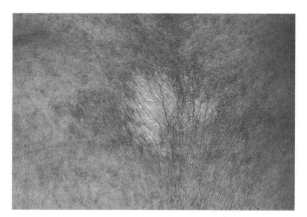

Fig. 26. Lichen sclerosus et atrophicus. White atrophic patch with wrinkling and peripheral erythema.

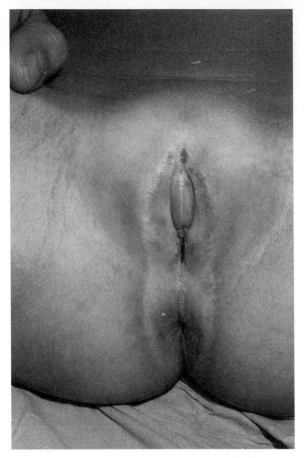

Fig. 27. Lichen sclerosus et atrophicus. Glistening white areas in the vulvar and perianal regions, creating a figure 8 or hourglass pattern. In the vulvar area there is more erythema, reflecting the pruritus and resultant excoriations.

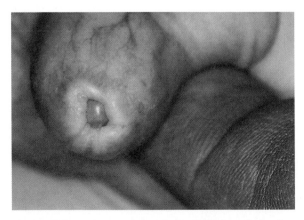

Fig. 28. Lichen sclerosus et atrophicus. Typical penile involvement with phimosis.

Symptoms

While extragenital disease is usually asymptomatic, the genital lesions may be pruritic or the patient may experience burning pain on urination.

Diagnosis

The diagnosis can easily be made clinically and a traumatic biopsy in a sensitive area is rarely needed. Some authors suggest screening for autoimmune disease, especially thyroid disease.

Differential Diagnosis

In the anogenital region, vitiligo is the most difficult differential diagnostic consideration, while on the trunk, there is a clinical overlap with morphea (Table 27). In some instances, these two diseases cannot be separated with certainty and some experts consider them as part of the same disease spectrum. Sexual abuse has to be kept in mind as a possibility when hemorrhage, bruising and erosions are present in the anogenital area.

Table 27. Differential diagnosis of lichen sclerosus et atrophicus

Diagnosis	Distinguishing Features
■ **Anogenital disease**	
Dermatitis	Erythema with scaling and without atrophy; marked pruritus
Vitiligo	Depigmentation without atrophy or pruritus; other body areas usually affected
Sexual abuse	Sudden onset, lack of pruritus, lack of atrophy, hymen never involved in LSA, but might be injured in sexual abuse
■ **Extragenital disease**	
Morphea	No follicular hyperkeratoses; lilac peripheral ring

Table 28. Therapeutic approach to anogenital LSA

Week	Treatment
1–4	High potency corticosteroid ointment b.i.d. with frequent application of non-medicated emollient ointment throughout the day May use wet compresses for 30 minutes b.i.d. after the application of corticosteroid or emollient As the erythema and pruritus improve, move to the next level
5–8	Corticosteroid only applied in the evening Continue the non-medicated emollient ointment as desired
After week 8	Continue basic care Use the corticosteroids either once weekly to once monthly as needed

Therapy

Extragenital lesions in children often resolve spontaneously and treatment is frequently unnecessary. Anogenital disease responds very well to mid- to high potency topical corticosteroids. There are reports of a sufficient response in boys to resolve a phimosis, making circumcision unnecessary. When circumcision is performed, the disease is surprisingly almost always cured in boys. The new topical macrolide immunosuppressants may present an alternative to corticosteroid treatment, thus, minimizing the risk of iatrogenic atrophy in a sensible area with high absorption where UV-induced photocarcinogenesis is not an issue (Table 28).

Patients and parents should be instructed about proper anogenital hygiene using soap substitutes if necessary, avoiding irritants and applying emollients on a regular basis.

Prognosis

There is no precise data about the prognosis of LSA in prepubertal girls. A substantial proportion seems to become free of symptoms at puberty, but at least 50% develop LSA in adult life. Often it is mild and may be overlooked or misdiagnosed.

References

Cruces M. J., De la Torre C., Losada A., Ocampo C., Garcia-Doval I.: Infantile pyramidal protrusion as a manifestation of lichen sclerosus et atrophicus. Arch Dermatol 134:1118–1120 (1998)

Dalziel K. L., Wojnarowska F.: Long-term control of vulval lichen sclerosus after treatment with a potent steroid cream. Journal of Reproductive Medicine 38:25–27 (1993)

Fischer G., Roger M.: Vulvar disease in children: a clinical audit of 130 cases. Pediatr Dermatol 17:1–6 (2000)

Garzon M. C., Paller A. S.: Ultrapotent topical corticosteroid treatment of childhood genital lichen sclerosus. Arch Dermatol 135:525-528 (1999)

Meuli M., Briner J., Hanimann B.: Lichen sclerosus et atrophicus causing phimosis in boys: a prospective study with 5-year follow-up after complete circumcision. Journal of Urology 152:987–989 (1994)

Powell J., Wojnarowska F.: Lichen sclerosus. Lancet 353:1777–1783 (1999)

Powell J., Wojnarowska F., Winsey S., Marren P., Welsh K.: Lichen sclerosus premenarche: autoimmunity and immunogenetics. Br J Dermatol 142: 481–484 (2000)

Turner M. L. C.: Management of lichen sclerosus. Current Opinion in Dermatology 3:3–9 (1996)

CHAPTER 12 Lyme Borreliosis

M. MÖHRENSCHLAGER

Epidemiology

Lyme borreliosis is a multi-systemic disease that can be caused by three different species of the *Borrelia burgdorferi sensu lato* complex: *B. afzelii, B. garinii, and B. sensu stricto*. In Europe, all three species can be found in patients with Lyme disease, where in the United States only *B. burgdorferi sensu stricto* plays a role in humans. Cases of Lyme borreliosis have been reported from all temperate regions of North America, Europe, and Asia. The main vector for the transfer of the organism in Europe is the tick *Ixodes ricinus*; in the United States primarily *Ixodes scapularis* and *Ixodes pacificus*. Ixodes develops in three stages – from larvae to nymph to adult tick. The ticks become infected by feeding on small mammals or certain birds which serve as reservoirs for *Borrelia burgdorferi*. In central Europe between 8–34% of *I. ricinus* have been found to carry *Borrelia burgdorferi*. Borrelia can be transmitted in any stage from infected parasites; the risk seems to be highest in nymphs as they are not readily removed due to their small size. While exact data is not available for Germany, as Lyme borreliosis is not a reportable disease, it is estimated that the risk of developing the disorder following a tick bite in endemic areas is 0.5–1.0%. The peak incidence rates are during the times when exposure to ticks is most common, from the late spring until well into autumn. More cases are seen in rural areas and especially suburban areas where there is a broad interface between dwelling areas and woods.

For the entire USA, the incidence of Lyme borreliosis was estimated as 6/100,000 in 1999. Clearly in endemic areas such as the Lyme river valley, the rate is dramatically higher. Children between 5 and 10 years of age as well as people with occupational or recreational exposure to tick-infested woods or fields are at greater risk of acquiring the disease.

Pathogenesis

Borrelia burgdorferi is a Gram-negative bacterium with 7–11 periplasmatic flagellae, growing preferably in a microaerophilic environment. The various subspecies differ in their antigenic profile (especially outer surface proteins, Osp A, Osp B, Osp C) and the spectrum of clinical manifestations. *Borrelia burgdorferi* is injected into the dermis by nymphal or adult ticks while feeding on human blood; the risk of transmission rises substantially with feeding times >24 hours. The bacteria spread in a centrifugal pattern in the connective tissue and often elicit a local reactive lymphocytic response. In some cases *Borrelia* enter into the systemic circulation at an early stage of disease causing flu-like symptoms. Usually hematogenous spread takes place weeks to months after the tick bite, with *Borrelia* accumulating preferentially in skin, synovia, central nervous system, eyes and heart. This may be followed by a chronic stage involving skin, joints or central nervous system. A humoral immune response is seen after 3–4 weeks (IgM) and 4–6 weeks (IgG) after infection, respectively.

Without treatment about 10% proceed from localized to disseminated disease and of these 10% to chronic disease.

Clinical Features

Lyme borreliosis is divided into three clinical stages, which frequently show overlaps.

■ **Early Localized Disease.** Following a tick bite and the transfer of *Borrelia burgdorferi*, after somewhere between 3 and 30 days, a small red to blue-red papule appears at the bite site. From this lesion develops a centrifugally spreading erythematous patch known as erythema migrans (Fig. 29). In about 80% of the patients, there is central clearing as the periphery advances producing an annular le-

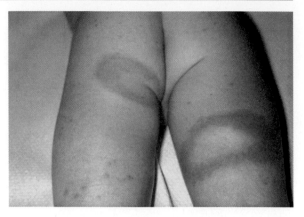

Fig. 30. Lyme borreliosis. Erythemata migrantia, or multiple lesions of erythema migrans on the thighs.

sion. These rings may become quite large, reaching 60 cm in diameter. Epidermal changes are uncommon. Sites of predilection are the legs in older children and adults, the head and neck in smaller children. In general, erythema migrans resolves spontaneous within two months, with a span of days to 14 months.

■ **Early Disseminated Disease.** The most common manifestation of early disseminated disease is multiple erythemata migrantia (Fig. 30), appearing a few weeks after the tick bite. A unilateral facial erythema in childhood, often with changing degrees of intensity, is also very suggestive of early disseminated Lyme borreliosis (Fig. 31). It is often overlooked because the complex features of the face make the annular pattern difficult to appreciate. Some patients experience flu-like signs and symptoms during this stage, including fever, headache, nuchal rigidity, myalgias, arthralgias, arthritis, and lymphadenopathy.

Weeks to months after the initial infection, another common cutaneous sign of Lyme borreliosis may appear: a red to red-brown nodule, usually solitary on the ear (Fig. 32) or nipple, or less often in the axillae, groin or dorsal aspect of the feet. These lesions are known as borrelial lymphocytoma or lymphadenosis cutis benigna (Bäfverstedt). Contrary to popular belief, they do

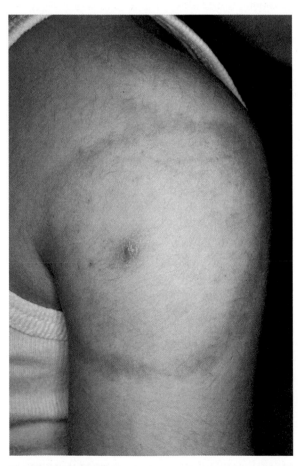

Fig. 29. Lyme borreliosis. Erythema migrans with peripheral annular erythema and central papule at site of initial tick bite.

lymphadenopathy. Other manifestations at this stage include nerve palsies (especially facial nerve palsy), radiculoneuritis, lymphocytic meningitis, carditis and eye involvement.

■ **Late Stage Disease.** In Europe the most common manifestation of late stage Lyme borreliosis is characterized by erythematous periarticular infiltrates which evolve into patches of strikingly thin skin (cigarette paper skin) with telangiectases and pigmentary changes, known as acrodermatitis chronica atrophicans. Such changes are extremely uncommon in children. In contrast, in the United States the most prevalent sign of chronic *Borrelia burgdorferi* infection is arthritis, usually monoarticular or oligoarticular involving large joints. Other extracutaneous late stage complications are mainly neurological such as encephalitis and polyneuropathy.

Symptoms

About 1/3 of patients with erythema migrans complain of pruritus. In other cases, they experience local warmth or burning. Some patients complain of fever, malaise, arthralgias, and other flu-like symptoms in early stage borreliosis. In late stage Lyme disease there is a wide variety of symptoms depending on which organ systems are involved.

Diagnosis

While the diagnosis of erythema migrans can usually be made clinically, the presence of Lyme borreliosis is confirmed by serological testing. Specific antibodies against *Borrelia burgdorferi* antigens are identified. The IgM antibodies first appear in the ELISA test about three weeks after the infection, so there is a window when the diagnosis cannot be confirmed serologically. By the time a borrelial lymphocytoma, arthritis or acro-

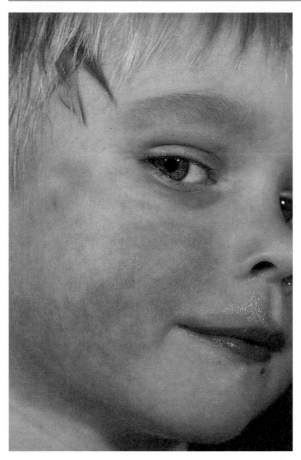

Fig. 31. Lyme borreliosis. Unilateral pale facial erythema with just a hint of an annular pattern.

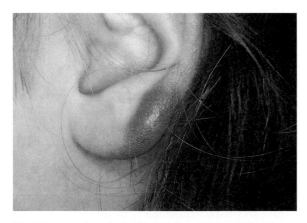

Fig. 32. Lyme borreliosis. Typical borrelial pseudolymphoma of ear lobe with livid red color.

not arise only at sites of tick bites. They typically resolve spontaneously, but may persist for many months or even several years. About 25% of individuals have an associated

Lyme Borreliosis

dermatitis chronica atrophicans develops, serological testing is always positive. Direct microscopic visualization is extremely difficult; culture and identification of *Borrelia burgdorferi* DNA by PCR are laborious procedures and not performed in routine practice. To minimize the risk of false-positive results (for example in rheumatic disease), confirmation of positive ELISA tests by Western blot is recommended. Of note, IgG antibodies persist over years and often life-long. In Western Europe, 10–15% of the population have IgG antibodies against *Borrelia burgdorferi* antigens. Elevated IgM antibodies may be detectable for months after acute infection and despite adequate treatment. Quite often IgM titers even rise during treatment, falling very slowly afterwards. If serological tests are performed, the time course of the production of IgM and IgG antibodies must be kept in mind. In addition, serological testing should be confined to patients with clinical signs and symptoms of the disease to avoid overdiagnosis and overtreatment. This situation is less of a problem in children.

Differential Diagnosis

The major differential diagnostic considerations for erythema migrans are shown in Table 29. Lymphadenosis cutis benigna must be distinguished from a persistent arthropod bite reaction (including nodular scabies), although these tend to be pruritic. In small children, a single mastocytoma can be mistaken for lymphadenosis cutis benigna, although it tends to be more brownish and urticate on manipulation (Darier sign). A cutaneous lymphoma is always in the histological differential diagnosis and may sometimes cause clinical confusion. Cutaneous B cell lymphoma in children usually presents with multiple lesions. In both arthropod bite reactions and B cell lymphomas, the borrelial serology should be negative.

Table 29. Differential diagnosis of erythema migrans

Diagnosis	Distinguishing Features
■ **Tinea corporis**	Peripheral scale; often multiple lesions; other family members affected; pets in household; pruritic; KOH and culture positive
■ **Erythema annulare centrifugum**	Peripheral scale; often more pruritic; multiple lesions more common; lesions more transient
■ **Erysipelas**	Peripheral confluent erythema with local warmth; fever, chills, lymphadenopathy; erythrocyte sedimentation rate ↑, WBC count ↑, positive streptococcal serology
■ **Erysipeloid**	Usually erythematous macule on hand in individual with contact with fresh meat or fish (butcher, hunter, fisherman)
■ **Fixed drug eruption**	Recurrent, often burning, lesion following ingestion of medication

Therapy

The acute Lyme borreliosis (early localized disease) should be treated with systemic antibiotics to eliminate *Borrelia burgdorferi* and thus remove the possibility of disease progression (Table 30). While the tetracyclines are the standard therapy is adults, they should not be used in children under 9 years of age because of teeth discoloration and enamel hypoplasia. In children, the agents of choice are amoxicillin or cefuroxime axetil. In the case of penicillin allergy, either erythromycin or azithromycin can be used. The duration of therapy should be 14 days, with the exceptions that erythromycin must be given for 21 days and azithromycin can be used for just 5–10 days. If the skin lesions or other signs and symptoms persist, the therapy should be extended for one week.

Early disseminated and late disease has traditionally been treated with intravenous ceftriaxone for 14 and 21, days, respectively. Intravenous cefotaxime and penicillin are alternatives. In cases with only cutaneous dis-

Table 30. Treatment of Lyme borreliosis

Medication	Total daily Dose	Route	Divided doses	Duration (days)[1]
■ **Early localized disease**				
■ **Early disseminated disease with cutaneous involvement only**				
Amoxicillin	50 mg/kg	p.o.	t.i.d.	14–21
Cefuroxime axetil	30 mg/kg	p.o.	b.i.d.	14–21
Erythromycin	40 mg/kg	p.o.	t.i.d.[2]	21
Azithromycin	10 mg/kg	p.o.	once[3]	5–10
Doxycycline[4]	200 mg	p.o.	b.i.d.[5]	14–21
Penicillin V	50,000 IU/kg	p.o.	t.i.d.[6]	14–21
■ **Early disseminated disease**				
Ceftriaxone	20–80 mg/kg	i.v.	once	14
Cefotaxime	50–100 mg/kg	i.v.	t.i.d.	14
Penicillin G	250,000 IU/kg	i.v.	q.i.d.	14
Amoxicillin[7]	50 mg/kg	p.o.	t.i.d.	30
Doxycycline[4,7]	200 mg	p.o.	b.i.d.[5]	30
■ **Late stage disease**				
Ceftriaxone	20–80 mg/kg	i.v.	once	21
Cefotaxime	50–100 mg/kg	i.v.	t.i.d.	21
Penicillin G	250,000 IU/kg	i.v.	q.i.d.	21
Amoxicillin[7]	50 mg/kg	p.o.	t.i.d.	21
Doxycycline[4,7]	200 mg	p.o.	b.i.d.[5]	30

i.v. intravenous; p.o. orally

[1] based on our experience; [2] with meals; [3] one hour before or 2 hours after meals; [4] not for children < 9 years of age; [5] give with adequate fluids or a meal; [6] one hour before meals; [7] with skin involvement only, in mild cases of Lyme arthritis, carditis or ophthalmologic disease with close follow-up

ease, it has now become accepted that oral amoxicillin or doxycycline (in older children) can be employed for pseudolymphoma, multiple erythemata migrantia and even acrodermatitis chronica atrophicans. When neurological disease is present, there is general agreement that intravenous treatment is mandatory, whereas in mild cases of Lyme arthritis, carditis or ophthalmic disease, oral treatment may be tried over a prolonged period of time, followed by intravenous therapy if unsuccessful. The Jarisch-Herxheimer reaction, well known in the treatment of syphilis, can also be seen during the first days of treating Lyme borreliosis, although it is usually much milder in Lyme borreliosis. Patients may experience fever, chills, an enhancement of the erythema migrans, malaise, headache, and radicular pain. Reactions are somewhat more common with penicillin, amoxicillin or doxycycline and less common with erythromycin. They resolve within a few days and are not an indication for discontinuing treatment. Non-steroidal anti-inflammatory drugs may help to alleviate symptoms.

Lyme Borreliosis

The prognosis for Lyme borreliosis in children is excellent. The typical cutaneous lesions allow early identification and prompt treatment, usually avoiding systemic complications. In the case of inadequate or absent therapy, a small percentage of patients will advance to have serious systemic diseases requiring more aggressive treatment.

Prophylaxis

Children playing or hiking in wooded areas should wear light-colored clothing, so that ticks can be more easily discovered. Long pants and long-sleeved shirts, as well as a closed collar and a baseball cap, offer additional protection. Ideally socks should be high enough so that they can be pulled up over the pants legs and closed shoes should be worn. The use of insect repellents sounds inviting but offers relatively little protection against ticks. In addition, many of the repellents are irritating, especially to the more sensitive skin of children. Thus, we do not recommend their use.

Since in almost all cases the transmission of *Borrelia burgdorferi* requires that the tick be attached to the host for more than 24 hours, a complete body check (not forgetting the scalp, face, ears and neck) should be performed every evening after possible exposure. If a tick is identified, it should be removed. While there are hundreds of methods recommended, simply grasping the ticket with a tweezers and gently extracting is usually sufficient. If the mouth parts are left behind, they will fall out by themselves. Techniques such as suffocating the tick with Vaseline, killing it with gasoline or burning it are obsolete and more likely to hurt the child than to facilitate removal.

The classic question is – should a child from whom a tick is removed in an a endemic area receive prophylactic antibiotics. The incidence of Lyme borreliosis is so low that in most cases, we do not recommend this approach. Parents should be instructed to look for erythema in the area of the tick bite during the following weeks and to seek medical care if there is anything suggestive of erythema migrans. The one exception is immunosuppressed children, where we generally prescribe amoxicillin. Testing the tick for borrelial infection is costly and of little predictive value for actual transmission of the disease.

An active immunization of children against *Borrelia burgdorferi* is possible and has been carried out in a few small study groups for children 2–15 years of age. A vaccine based on the recombinant surface protein OspA is approved in the USA for individuals 15 years of age or older. The side effects include pain at the injection site, myalgias, fever, chills, and headache, all of which resolve rapidly within a few days. While the immunization can be recommended in the USA, it is only effective for *Borrelia burgdorferi sensu stricto* and does not protect against *Borrelia garinii* and *Borrelia afzelii*, the other common European species which have different OspA antigens. Preclinical testing in Europe is underway using recombinant OspC and other possible agents.

References

American Academy of Pediatrics. Committee on Infectious Diseases: Prevention of Lyme disease. Pediatrics 105:142–147 (2000)

Anonymus. CDC Lyme WHO-CC. *http://www.cdc.gov*

Arnez M., Radsel-Medvescek A., Pleterski-Rigler D., Ruzic-Sabljic E., Strle F.: Comparison of cefuroxime axetil and phenoxymethyl penicillin for the treatment of children with solitary erythema migrans. Wiener Klinische Wochenschrift 111:916–922 (1999)

Beran J., de Clercq N., Dieussaert I., van Hoecke C.: Reactogenicity and immunogenicity of a Lyme disease vaccine in children 2–5 years old. Clinical Infectious Diseases 31:1504–1507 (2000)

Centers for Disease Control and Prevention: Lyme disease – United States, 1999. Journal of the American Medical Association 285:1698–1699 (2001)

Feder H.M.: Pitfalls in the diagnosis and treatment of Lyme disease in children. Journal of the American Medical Association 274:66–68 (1995)

Feder H.M., Beran J., van Hoecke C., Abraham B., de Clercq N., Buscarino C., Parenti D.L.: Immunogenicity of a recombinant *Borrelia burgdor*-

feri outer surface protein A vaccine against Lyme disease in children. Journal of Pediatrics 135: 575–579 (1999)

Klein J.O.: History of macrolide use in pediatrics. Pediatric Infectious Diseases Journal 16:427–431 (1997)

Oschmann P., Kraiczy P., Halperin J., Brade V. (eds): Lyme Borreliosis and Tick-borne Encephalitis. Unimed, Bremen (1999)

Paul H., Gerth H.J., Ackermann R.: Infectiousness for humans of *Ixodes ricinus* containing *Borrelia burgdorferi.* Zentralblatt für Bakteriologie und Hygiene (A) 263:473–476 (1986)

Piesman J., Mather T.N., Sinsky R.J., Spielman A.: Duration of tick attachment and *Borrelia burgdorferi* transmission. Journal of Clinical Microbiology 25:557–558 (1987)

Salazaar J.C., Gerber M.A., Goff C.W.: Long-term outcome of Lyme disease in children given early treatment. The Journal of Pediatrics 122:591–593 (1993)

Shapiro E.D., Gerber M.A.: Lyme disease. Clinical Infectious Diseases 31:533–542 (2000)

Sigal L.H., Zahradnik J.M., Lavin P., Patella S.J., Bryant G., Haselby R., Hilton E., Kunkel M., Adler-Klein D., Doherty T., Evans J., Malawista S.E., and the recombinant outer surface protein A Lyme disease vaccine study consortium: A vaccine consisting of recombinant *Borrelia burgdorferi* outer-surface protein A to prevent Lyme disease. New England Journal of Medicine 339:216–222 (1998)

Steere A.C., Sikand V.K., Meurice F., Parenti D.L., Fikrig E., Schoen R.T., Nowakowski J., Schmid C.H., Laukamp S., Buscarino C., Krause D.C., and the Lyme disease vaccine study group: Vaccination against Lyme disease with recombinant *Borrelia burgdorferi* outer-surface lipoprotein A with adjuvant. New England Journal of Medicine 339:209–215 (1998)

Weber K., Pfister H.W.: Clinical management of Lyme borreliosis. Lancet 343:1017–1020 (1994)

CHAPTER 13 Cutaneous Mastocytosis

K. Brockow

Epidemiology

The incidence of cutaneous mastocytosis is unknown. Perhaps 1 in every 8–10,000 dermatology patients has some form of mastocytosis. About 55% of cases appear in the first two years of life and over 2/3 begin in childhood. The disorder is usually sporadic with no genetic predisposition, although about 50 cases of familial mastocytosis have been described.

Pathogenesis

Mastocytosis is characterized by a proliferation of mast cells. In the skin, mast cells are normally located about blood vessels and when stimulated either by immunologic or non-immunologic mechanisms release a variety of mediators. In adults, cutaneous mast cell infiltrates may be associated with a systemic proliferation of malignant mast cells (mast cell leukemia), but in children this is almost never the case. Both local excess production of mast cell growth factors as well as aberrant mast cell surface receptors could explain the mast cell hyperplasia.

The cause of mast cell disease in children is unknown. In adults somatic mutation in the KIT gene, the receptor for stem cell factor, is often the cause of the disease. While a variety of mutations have been found in children, their clinical relevance is unclear. The signs and symptoms of mast cell disease can be explained by the increased number of cells and

their excessive production and release of mediators. Histamine, neutral proteases and proteoglycans are stored in mast cell granules and released on stimulation. In addition, a variety of lipid mediators (prostaglandin D2, sulfidoleukotriene and platelet activating factor [PAF]) are immediately synthesized and released. This barrage of mediators causes vasodilatation, increased vessel permeability, and smooth muscle contraction which can lead to anaphylactic reactions. Mast cell cytokines probably cause the many systemic symptoms which bedevil patients.

Clinical Features

There are several different clinical variants of mastocytosis. The most common is urticaria pigmentosa, which is a maculopapular cutaneous eruption. Clinically one sees red-brown macules and minimally raised papules (Fig. 33). The lesions vary in size from a few mm to several cm. The lesions are irregularly distributed but usually widespread; the trunk and thighs are most commonly affected, while the palms and soles are usually spared. Urticaria pigmentosa is a misnomer, in that the lesions are not true urticaria, are only lightly pigmented but more telangiectatic. When a lesion of urticaria pigmentosa is manipulated, the mast cells may degranulate and then cause an urticarial lesion; this response is known as Darier sign.

The other common form of mast cell disease in children is a solitary mastocytoma. Here one or more raised, red-brown papules are present; on occasion they evolve into large nodules or plaques (Abb. 34). On occasion, the lesions may develop bullae (Abb. 35). Darier sign is once again positive and not all lesions are pigmented.

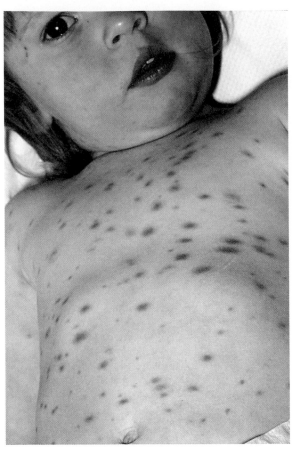

Fig. 33. Urticaria pigmentosa with disseminated red-brown macules on trunk.

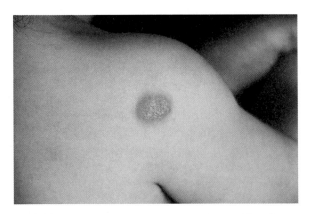

Fig. 34. Solitary mastocytoma presenting as yellow-brown nodule on shoulder.

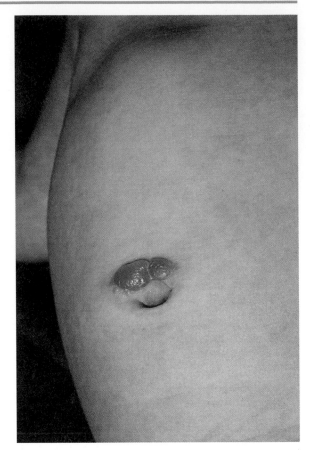

Fig. 35. Solitary mastocytoma with two tense overlying blisters filled with yellow-brown fluid near the umbilicus.

Diffuse cutaneous mastocytosis is an uncommon but very dramatic clinical picture. It almost always appears in infancy. The skin is diffusely swollen and has a dough-like consistency with an orange skin surface pattern. In addition, it may have varying shades of red, yellow, and brown. In early childhood, the intense edema usually leads to the spontaneous formation of blisters, but this alarming tendency resolves spontaneously. The blisters are tense and hemorrhagic, but heal without significant scarring. In some infants, blisters are the first clinical sign, so mastocytosis must always be considered in the differential diagnosis of childhood bullous diseases. These same children may be at risk for dramatic gastrointestinal reactions with shock and hemorrhage. Systemic involvement of the bone marrow, gastrointestinal tract, spleen, liver or lymph nodes is most rare in children.

The local release of heparin in the skin may also lead to prolonged cutaneous bleeding following trauma or even minor medical intervention, such as a skin biopsy. In the same vein, severe anaphylactic reactions (dyspnea, tachycardia, syncope, shock) have been described following arthropod assaults and administration of mast cell degranulators in adults; children with diffuse disease should be watched for similar problems.

Symptoms

The only significant symptom in children is pruritus. Mechanical irritation (rough or tightly fitting clothing), warmth (hot shower or bath), physical activity or sudden changes in temperature (diving into cold water) can produce a flare of the skin lesions with dramatic pruritus and sometimes systemic signs and symptoms. In a study of 17 children with mastocytosis, 65% reported flushing; 41%, gastrointestinal problems such as pain, vomiting or diarrhea; 18%, headache; and 12%, bone pain.

Diagnosis

The diagnosis can usually be made clinically; the typical red-brown color and the positive Darier sign are reliable clues. A skin biopsy can confirm the diagnosis. When a papule or nodule is biopsied, the mast cells can be seen easily with H&E stain, but when more diffuse or macular disease is present, a toluidine blue, Giemsa or tryptase stain is very helpful. Serum tryptase levels of >20 ng/mL suggest systemic involvement. Further diagnostic measures are only indicated when systemic involvement is suspected.

Table 31. Differential diagnostic considerations for mast cell disease

Diagnosis	Distinguishing Features
Urticarial lesions	
■ Urticaria	Transient lesions; no persistent lesions; no pigmentary changes; dermographism on clinically normal skin
■ Persistent arthropod bite or sting reaction	Intensely pruritic papules; no pigmentary changes; slow resolution
Nodules	
■ Juvenile xanthogranuloma	Red-yellow papules and nodules; often scalp; non-pruritic; Darier sign negative; also resolve spontaneously; often only distinguishable with histologic examination
■ Spitz nevus	Persistent red-brown papule; usually solitary; non-pruritic; Darier sign negative; often only distinguishable with histologic examination
Pigmented lesions	
Multiple lentigines or ephelides (freckles)	Many smaller pigmented lesions; non-pruritic; Darier sign negative; may be associated with photosensitivity or a variety of syndromes
Pigmented lichen planus	Pigmented macules following pruritic eruption; tend to fade with time; Darier sign negative

Differential Diagnosis

Table 31 shows the differential diagnostic considerations which should be entertained.

Therapy

The therapeutic approach to mast cell disease is shown in Table 32.

■ **General Measures.** A curative approach to cutaneous mast cell disease is not available. The symptomatic treatment must be tailored

Table 32. Treatment of mast cell disease

■ **General measures**	Counseling Avoidance of degranulating events and agents
■ **Watchful waiting**	Appropriate if pruritus absent or tolerable
■ **Oral antihistamines**	Non-sedating agents such as levocetirizine or desloratadine; if pruritus persists, combine with sedating agent in the evening; if gastrointestinal symptoms, use H2 blocker (cimetidine)
■ **Mast cell stabilizers**	Cromolyn if gastrointestinal symptoms are present
■ **Phototherapy**	UVA1 or PUVA for marked pruritus
■ **Topical corticosteroids**	Useful for highly pruritic or bullous lesions

to each patient in an individual manner. The patient and/or parents should be made aware of the generally benign nature of childhood mast cell disease and be informed about potential mast cell degranulators which often worsen the condition. Included in the list are physical stimuli (mechanical stimulation, heat, cold, exercise), medications (acetylsalicylic acid, opiates such as morphine and codeine, polymyxin B, x-ray contrast materials) and arthropod bites and stings. Patients with widespread disease or cardiovascular symptoms should carry an emergency kit containing an antihistamine solution, prednisolone suppository and epinephrine spray. If the child requires surgery, the anesthesiologist should be informed well in advance of the presence of mast cell disease, even though in most instances no problems are encountered.

■ **Systemic Therapy.** Oral antihistamines are the mainstay in treating the almost inevitable pruritus associated with mast cell disease (see Appendix III). We recommend non-sedating agents such as levocetirizine or desloratadine; usually twice daily administration suffices. If the non-sedating agents are

not effective, we switch to an older sedating agent such as dimethindene maleate or hydroxyzine liquid. In most children, drowsiness occurs but is a surmountable problem. A useful plan is to combine a sedating agent in the evening with a non-sedating one in the morning. Another possibility is to combine a non-sedating agent with an H2 blocker (cimetidine 200 mg daily); this is especially useful if gastrointestinal symptoms are present.

Another approach is to use mast cell degranulation inhibitors. Ketotifen is both a granule stabilizer and H1 blocker; however in one study, it was not more effective than hydroxyzine. Oral cromolyn (20–40 mg/kg daily) may be useful for gastrointestinal disease, but is not absorbed enough to reach cutaneous mast cells. Cromolyn must be taken q.i.d. and regularly; otherwise the mast cells escape the blockage.

Phototherapy with UVA1 or PUVA leads to moderate improvement in the cutaneous symptoms which lasts for a surprisingly long period of time, but in view of its long-term side effects, we rarely use phototherapy in infants or small children with a generally self-limited disease.

Systemic corticosteroids are only rarely used, and then for severe bullous disease. Bolus therapy with methylprednisolone (1 mg/kg in a single daily dose for one or several days) can arrest bullous disease.

■ **Topical Therapy.** High-potency topical corticosteroids are effective for short-term control of intensely pruritic or bullous skin lesions. They should be used 1–2 times daily, perhaps under occlusion, for several days to a week. Blisters can be punctured, drained, and then treated with a topical antiseptic or a less potent corticosteroid cream such as mometasone fuorate.

Prognosis

The outlook for cutaneous mastocytosis in children is good. Often the skin is the only involved organ; systemic disease is most uncommon. In over 50% of cases, and in almost all mastocytomas, the disease has resolved by puberty. Those rare children with diffuse cutaneous mastocytosis and systemic involvement have a more varied outlook. In some, the disease persists into adult life but in most cases takes a mild course and does not influence their life expectancy.

References

Brockow K., Metcalfe D. D.: Mastocytosis, pp 55.1–55.9. In: Rich, Fleisher T. R., Shearer W. T., Kotzin B. L., Schroeder H. W. (eds) Clinical Immunology – Principles and Practice. Mosby International Ltd, London, Edinburgh, New York, Volume 1 (2001)

Hartmann K., Metcalfe D. D.: Pediatric mastocytosis. Hematol Oncol Clin North Am 14:625–640 (2000)

Heide R., Tank B., Oranje A. P.: Mastocytosis in childhood. Ped Dermatol 19:375–381 (2002)

Kettelhut B. V., Metcalfe D. D.: Pediatric mastocytosis. Ann Allergy 73:197–202 (1994)

Longley J., Duffy P. T., Kohn S.: The mast cell and mast cell disease. J Am Acad Dermatol 32:545–561 (1995)

CHAPTER 14 Molluscum Contagiosum

K. BROCKOW

Epidemiology

Mollusca contagiosa are a worldwide problem, most commonly found in children, especially patients with atopic dermatitis and those who are immunosuppressed. Warm moist climates and poor personal hygiene lead to an increased frequency of infection.

Pathogenesis

The molluscum contagiosum virus is a member of the pox virus family. It is exclusively epidermotropic. The incubation period following transfer to the skin is short (14–50 days). In children the virus is transmitted by direct contact, such as during play or among siblings; in adults sexual activity is the most likely method of transfer. The decreased barrier function in patients with atopic dermatitis is felt to explain their susceptibility, while immunosuppressed patients produce less of an immune response to the attacking virus.

Clinical Features

The clinical features of mollusca contagiosa are distinctive – the individual lesion is a skin-colored to white firm 3–5 mm papule with a central dell. Usually multiple lesions are present (Fig. 36). The most common sites are the trunk and extremities. In patients with HIV/AIDS and other types of immunosuppression, extremely large lesions, often greater than 15 mm (mollusca conta-

giosa gigantea) can form. Solitary or stalked lesions are also seen. Sometimes there is irritation and a resultant erythema.

The course is difficult to predict. Spontaneous remission within 6–9 months is the rule, but this is a long period of time during which the lesions can be transmitted to other body parts or to other individuals. More lesions and less likelihood of spontaneous remission are features of those patients with atopic dermatitis or immunosuppression. Complications include enormous numbers of lesions, development of an associated dermatitis, secondary impetiginization or cellulitis surrounding a lesion, and intraorbital involvement.

Symptoms

The lesions are almost always asymptomatic. Some children experience marked pruritus, followed by excoriations and secondary in-

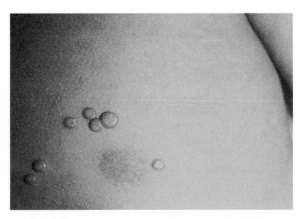

Fig. 36. Mollusca contagiosa. Multiple pale papules with central dells located about the nipple.

fections. The latter scenario is more common in atopic dermatitis patients.

Diagnosis

The diagnosis is clinical. If there are any questions, molluscum contagiosum virus produces a spectacular histologic picture with giant multi-colored inclusion bodies, allowing a rapid microscopic diagnosis.

Differential Diagnosis

The major differential diagnostic considerations are shown in Table 33.

Therapy

■ **Active Non-intervention/No Intervention.** Even though the spontaneous cure rate in mollusca contagiosa is high, it is impossible to predict the course in any given child. In some instances it may be appropriate to do nothing. We still usually try to have a "therapy plan" to take advantage of the placebo effect. Possibilities include pseudo-radiation therapy (without ionizing radiation), trivial doses of light, touching the lesions with nail polish, occluding them with tape or painting

Table 33. Differential diagnosis of mollusca contagiosa

Diagnosis	Distinguishing Features
■ **Juvenile papular dermatitis (sandbox dermatitis)**	Special form of atopic dermatitis with small firm papules without central dells; limited to knees, elbows
■ **Plane warts**	Flat topped papules; usually smaller than mollusca; often on face
■ **Skin tag**	Stalked lesion, often in axillae or on nape
■ **Dermatofibroma**	Usually solitary papule on leg with red-brown color and firm consistency
■ **Adenoma sebaceum**	Multiple red-yellow central facial papules in tuberous sclerosis

Table 34. Treatment of mollusca contagiosa

■ **Active non-intervention**
- occlusion
- pseudo-radiation therapy
- pseudo-light therapy
- painting with gentian violet
- improved skin care

■ **Curettage following EMLA**

■ **Squeezing**

■ **Cryotherapy**

■ **Other measures**
- salicylic acid plasters
- topical retinoids
- laser destruction
- 5% KOH solution
- imiquimod

them with a dye such as 0.25% aqueous gentian violet. If the child has dry skin or atopic dermatitis, increased skin care to restore the barrier function is also necessary (Table 34).

■ **Curettage.** Simple curettage is the standard treatment for mollusca contagiosa. While adults can almost always tolerate removal without anesthesia, in children we routinely employ EMLA (eutectic mixture of 2.5% lidocaine and 2.5% prilocaine). It is applied 1–2 hours prior to treatment under occlusive dressing (there are special non-permeable dressings, but simple plastic kitchen wrap or cellophane tape works just as well for single lesions). Because of the risk of systemic absorption (and subsequent induction of methemoglobinemia), EMLA should not be used in children receiving other methemoglobin-inducing drugs and special care must be taken in children with an impaired skin barrier. The maximum dosage given by the manufacturer are 1 g of EMLA in infants <3 months or <5 kg, 2 g in infants 3–12 months >5 kg, 10 g in children 1 to 10 years >10 kg, and 20 g in children 7–12 years >20 kg.

The tolerance of the child can also be improved by an attractive operating room atmosphere with appropriate distractions (toys, music). In addition, a sharp curette and stretching the skin taut during scraping greatly reduce pain. After popping off the molluscum body, the lesion is painted with 0.25% aqueous gentian violet or another antiseptic.

In patients with many lesions (>50), in sensitive regions (genitalia, periorbital) or in anxious children (often because of an ineffective and unsuccessful previous therapeutic attempt), it may be necessary to perform the curettage under general anesthesia.

■ **Squeezing.** Classic, non-inflamed mollusca can be treated by simply squeezing out the central keratotic plug with a fine curved forceps. This method has little risk of scarring, but does not work with all types of mollusca.

■ **Cryotherapy.** While cryotherapy may also work to destroy mollusca, it has many disadvantages and we do not often employ or recommend it. Without question, cryotherapy is much more painful and thus less suited for multiple lesions or repeat treatments. In addition, the frozen lesions become necrotic and drop off over a period of time, during which they may be painful or otherwise bother the child. Often the initial freeze is not successful and then multiple attempts are needed.

■ **Other Measures.** There are many other destructive measures which also can be employed, although we see little advantage except for more cost or more pain; included in this list are pulsed CO_2 and dye lasers, as well as electrocautery.

Both salicylic acid (usually as an impregnated plaster) and topical retinoids can be applied to mollusca. The resultant irritation often leads first to inflammation and then disappearance of the lesions. Another form of irritation is painting the lesions with 5–10% KOH solution once or twice daily for 4–6 weeks.

The topical immunomodulatory agent imiquimod (Aldara®) has also been used in the treatment of mollusca contagiosa with moderate response rates (30–53% complete clearance after 4–16 weeks), although it is not approved for usage in children. In published protocols, the imiquimod is applied once daily 3–7 times a week. The 5% preparation causes significant irritation, but the limiting practical factor appears to be its cost.

References

Gottlieb S. L., Myskowski P. L.: Molluscum contagiosum. International Journal of Dermatology 33: 453–461 (1994)

Hengge U. R., Esser S., Schultewolter T., Behrendt C., Meyer T., Stockfleth E., Goos M.: Self-administered topical 5% imiquimod for the treatment of common warts and molluscum contagiosum. Br J Dermatol 143:1026–1031 (2000)

Liota E., Smith K. J., Buckley R., Menon P., Skelton H.: Imiquimod therapy for molluscum contagiosum. J Cutan Med Surg 4:76–82 (2000)

Romiti R., Ribeiro A. P., Grimblat B. M., Rivitti E. A., Romiti N.: Treatment of molluscum contagiosum with potassium hydroxide: a clinical approach in 35 children. Pediatric Dermatology 16:228–231 (1999)

Siegfried E. C.: Warts and molluscum on children – an approach to therapy. Dermatological Therapy 2:51–67 (1997)

Skinner R. B. Jr, Ray S., Talanin N. Y.: Treatment of molluscum contagiosum with topical 5% imiquimod cream. Pediatr Dermatol 17:420 (2000)

CHAPTER 15 Perioral Dermatitis

K. STROM

Epidemiology

Although perioral dermatitis was first described in young adult women, it is also a common disease of childhood. Once again, girls are more often involved than boys. There appears to be an occasional association with atopic dermatitis.

Pathogenesis

The most important aspect of the pathogenesis is the use of potent topical corticosteroids on the face. Usually the history reveals that the patient has used these agents for a long time. In children, even hydrocortisone products may on occasion evoke perioral dermatitis. Occasionally perioral dermatitis has been observed in children using inhaled corticosteroids for asthma. Other possible triggers include fluoridated toothpastes and mouth washes, as well as the use of occlusive or greasy facial creams.

Clinical Features

The classic clinical picture of perioral dermatitis is grouped erythematous papules and papulo-vesicles about the mouth which typically do not extend to the vermilion border of the lip (Figs. 37 and 38). Similar lesions may be found in perinasal and periocular locations (Fig. 39). A granulomatous variant of perioral dermatitis has been described primarily in black children under the name of facial Afro-Caribbean eruption.

Symptoms

The lesions are usually asymptomatic. On occasion pruritus is described.

Diagnosis

The diagnosis can be made clinically; the key step is to search for an exposure to topical corticosteroids.

Differential Diagnosis

The major differential diagnostic considerations are shown in Table 35. Just as in adults, the most difficult distinction is between rosacea and perioral dermatitis. The situation is easier in children, as rosacea is

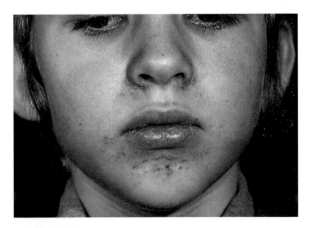

Fig. 37. Perioral dermatitis. Scattered red papules and papulo-vesicles in perioral and perinasal distribution with typical Grenz zone.

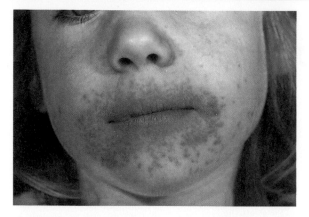

Fig. 38. Perioral dermatitis. More severe confluent involvement.

Table 35. Differential diagnosis of perioral dermatitis

Diagnosis	Distinguishing Features
■ **Rosacea**	Telangiectases; possible ocular involvement
■ **Seborrheic dermatitis**	Oily scales; involvement of seborrheic areas; lack of papules
■ **Atopic dermatitis**	Positive family history; patches of dermatitis elsewhere; pruritus
■ **Acne infantum or acne vulgaris**	Comedones

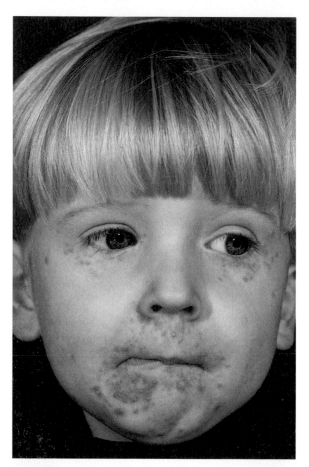

Fig. 39. Perioral dermatitis. Perioral, perinasal and periorbital papules and papulo-vesicles.

extremely rare. Fortunately the distinction is not crucial, as the treatment is identical. Seborrheic dermatitis is greasier, with scales predominating rather than papules and typi-

cally involves the scalp line. Atopic dermatitis is seldom so papular and usually involves other body areas at the same time. Acne infantum or acne vulgaris is often the initial diagnosis, but a careful search reveals the absence of comedones. Granulomatous perioral dermatitis shares many features with sarcoidosis; the diagnosis is made on the absence of systemic disease and the prompt response to therapy.

Therapy

Treatment involves stopping the use of topical corticosteroids and then trying to speed the spontaneous but slow resolution of the process. The single most important fact is that *the eruption will get worse* when topical corticosteroids are stopped. The physician must beg the parents and the patient not to restart corticosteroids, but instead to follow the outlined treatment (Table 36).

In adults, the easiest way to ameliorate this flare and facilitate the healing process is systemic tetracyclines. Since they are not recommended for children less than 9 years of age, topical antibiotics are the answer. The two most commonly employed agents are metronidazole and erythromycin. While metronidazole is more effective, it is not approved for perioral dermatitis or for childhood use. The role of metronidazole appears to be anti-inflammatory and immunosuppressive, rather than anti-microbial.

Table 36. Treatment of perioral dermatitis

■ Definitive therapy	**Stop topical corticosteroids!** Also discontinue fluoridated toothpastes and mouth washes, as well as occlusive facial products
■ Supportive therapy	Topical metronidazole (0.75–1% gel or oil-in-water emulsion); initially once daily; if tolerated, increase to b.i.d. As an alternative, topical erythromycin (1–2%) used in same way. Wet compresses if initially markedly inflamed or pruritic.

In many countries, metronidazole gel (0.75%) is available as a commercial product either as gel or as cream. If it is not available, we have had good luck compounding 1–2% metronidazole in an oil-in-water emulsion (water-based cream). We start out treating once daily and if the patient appears to be tolerating the product, we increase to b.i.d. application after 1 week. Often during the first week with the inevitable flare, cold compresses with tap water in addition to applying the medication are useful. Some patients find the gel too drying and require the cream. The patient should also use only one skin care product (to avoid skipping back and forth which is so common) and it should be a water-based cream. Occlusive products may play a triggering role and should be avoided.

As an alternative, a variety of topical erythromycin products are available. Most are solutions, but gels and even a cream are available. In addition, a 1–2% erythromycin base solution can be mixed in a similar vehicle as metronidazole. The product is used in exactly the same way.

Significant improvement is first seen after 4–6 weeks, and it may take 3–6 months to obtain a complete remission. As soon as there is a marked diminution of the inflammation and papules, one can cut back, using the topical metronidazole or erythromycin once daily in the evening or even once very other evening. We prefer to treat the patient for several months, rather than stopping as soon as improvement is seen, as rebound flares may occur when topical antibiotics are stopped.

References

Boeck K., Abeck D., Werfel S., Ring J.: Perioral dermatitis in children – clinical presentation, pathogenesis-related factors and response to topical metronidazole. Dermatology 195:235–238 (1997)

Cotterill J. A.: Perioral dermatitis. British Journal of Dermatology 101:259–262 (1979)

Frieden I. J., Prose N. S., Fletcher V., Turner M. L.: Granulomatous perioral dermatitis in children. Archives of Dermatology 125:369–373 (1989)

Laude T. A., Salvemini J. N.: Perioral dermatitis in children. Semin Cutan Med Surg 18:206–209 (1999)

Malik R., Quirk C. J.: Topical applications and perioral dermatitis. Australas J Dermatol 41:34–38 (2000)

Manders S. M., Lucky A. W.: Perioral dermatitis in childhood. Journal of the American Academy of Dermatology 27:688–692 (1992)

Miller S. R., Shalita A. R.: Topical metronidazole gel (0.75%) for the treatment of perioral dermatitis in children. Journal of the American Academy of Dermatology 31:847–848 (1994)

Savin J. A., Alexander S., Marks R.: A rosacea-like eruption of children. British Journal of Dermatology 87:425 (1972)

Wilkinson D. S., Kirton V., Wilkinson J. D.: Perioral dermatitis: a 12-year review. British Journal of Dermatology 101:245–257 (1979)

Perioral Dermatitis

C. Schnopp, T. Schmidt

Epidemiology

Little is available on the incidence of pityriasis lichenoides. It is typically a disease of children and young adults, affecting both sexes equally.

Pathogenesis

The cause of pityriasis lichenoides is unknown. The sudden appearance and resolution suggest a viral trigger, while the basic tissue reaction is one of vasculitis.

Clinical Features

There are two distinct stages of pityriasis lichenoides. The acute stage is known as pityriasis lichenoides et varioliformis acuta (PLEVA) or Mucha-Habermann disease. The classic lesions are erythematous papules which often have hemorrhage and central necrosis (Fig. 40). They favor the trunk and proximal extremities. The lesions appear suddenly, progress for a few days to weeks and then resolve spontaneously, leaving behind varioliform (resembling smallpox) scars.

The chronic stage is designated pityriasis lichenoides chronica. Here the lesions are less dramatic, appearing as small minimally inflamed papules with a thick scale (known in German as *Oblaten* scale, named after the sacramental wafers). When the scale is pulled off, a hypo- or hyperpigmented macule is left behind (Fig. 41). They favor the same body regions. The lesions of pityriasis lichenoides chronica may persist for years.

The presence of individuals with both types of lesions is taken as proof that the two diseases are related. Most patients with pityriasis lichenoides et varioliformis acuta do not go on to pityriasis lichenoides chronica; some with clear pityriasis lichenoides chronica do not give a convincing history of pityriasis lichenoides et varioliformis acuta (Fig. 42).

Symptoms

The amazing thing about pityriasis lichenoides et varioliformis acuta is that it looks terrible but is strikingly asymptomatic. On rare occasions, patients describe fever and malaise at the onset of their illness, lending support to the viral theory of origin.

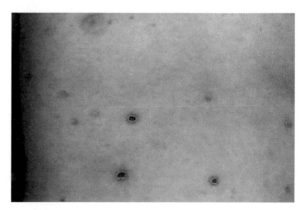

Fig. 40. Pityriasis lichenoides et varioliformis acuta. Disseminated eruption with multiple red papules as well as more infiltrated lesions with hemorrhage and central necrosis.

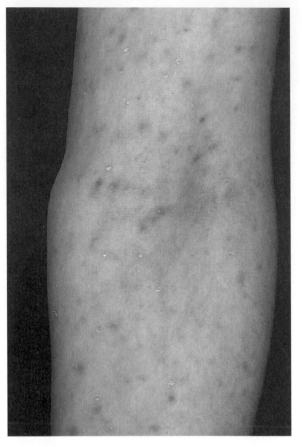

Fig. 41. Pityriasis lichenoides chronica. Multiple minimally erythematous papules, some with a central scale.

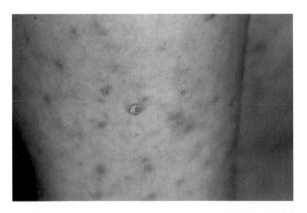

Fig. 42. Pityriasis lichenoides with transition from acute lesions of pityriasis lichenoides et varioliformis acuta to thick scales of pityriasis lichenoides chronica.

Diagnosis

The diagnosis is made clinically. In difficult cases, a skin biopsy may be helpful. There are no specific laboratory tests.

Differential Diagnosis

The major differential diagnostic considerations are shown in Table 37. An additional problem is lymphomatoid papulosis. This uncommon disease is almost unheard of in children under 10 years of age. It clinically resembles pityriasis lichenoides et varioliformis acuta but the lesions are usually larger and fewer in number. Microscopically they show striking lymphocytic atypia with the abnormal cells marking heavily for CD30. The course of lymphomatoid papulosis is one of recurrent lesions, with progression into lymphoma in perhaps 10% of cases.

Therapy

Most parents and children are agreeable to watchful neglect, once the nature of the peculiar eruption is explained to them. A limited number of lesions can be treated with a mid-potency topical corticosteroid (Table 38).

In the case of disseminated disease, the child may suffer both from their appearance

Table 37. Differential diagnosis of pityriasis lichenoides

Diagnosis	Distinguishing Features
■ **Lichen planus**	Violaceous flat-topped papules, especially about wrists, without hemorrhage or necrosis; pruritic
■ **Pityriasis rosea**	Oval lesions with collarette scale following skin line; often herald patch
■ **Guttate psoriasis**	Positive family history for psoriasis; antecedent streptococcal pharyngitis; involvement of face and scalp; pruritic; no hemorrhage

Table 38. Treatment of pityriasis lichenoides

■ **Watchful neglect**	Often no treatment is needed other than reassurance
■ **Topical corticosteroids**	Mid-potency corticosteroids can be applied once daily (in evening) to lesions
■ **Phototherapy**	Either UVB phototherapy or a several week vacation in a sunny area may help
■ **Macrolide antibiotics**	Either erythromycin for 4–8 weeks or roxithromycin for 2 weeks can be tried, especially if the patient has had prodromal signs and symptoms

and the taunting of their peers. In such cases, sunlight exposure or phototherapy is reasonable. Often the family can be encouraged to simply take a vacation for several weeks in a sunny climate. Either UVB or narrow spectrum (311 nm) UVB therapy over a time period of 4–6 weeks is helpful. In some instances, erythromycin or other macrolide antibiotics are given. It is most difficult to assess either of these approaches objectively, since they produce results over the same time period in which spontaneous resolution occurs.

A dramatic response can be seen with low-dose methotrexate, but its range of side effects generally prohibits its use for a benign disease in children.

References

Gelmetti C., Rigoni C., Alessi E., Ermacora E., Berti E., Caputo R.: Pityriasis lichenoides in children: a long-term follow-up of eighty-nine cases. Journal of the American Academy of Dermatology 23:473–478 (1990)

Romani J., Puig L., Fernandez-Figueras M., de Moragas J.M.: Pityriasis lichenoides in children: clinicopathologic review of 22 patients. Pediatric Dermatology 15:1–6 (1998)

Truhan A.P., Herbert A.A., Esterly N.B.: Pityriasis lichenoides in children: therapeutic response to erythromycin. Journal of the American Academy of Dermatology 15:66–70 (1986)

Pityriasis Lichenoides

CHAPTER 17

Pityriasis Rosea

M. MÖHRENSCHLAGER

Epidemiology

Pityriasis rosea is a common self-limited papulo-squamous disorder which accounts for about 2% of the patients in a dermatology practice. Although the disease can occur in every age group, it favors children and young adults. Females may be slightly more often affected. Characteristic is the occurrence of pityriasis rosea in clusters, more often in the spring and fall.

Pathogenesis

The cause of pityriasis rosea is unknown. A viral etiology appears most likely and human herpes virus has been suggested as the most likely candidate, but the association is not well-proven. Other postulated etiologies that seem less likely include autoimmune reactions, psychological factors and in some rare cases, medications or exposure to toxins. Gold salts for example produce a pityriasis rosea-like eruption, but most patients are adults with rheumatoid arthritis.

Clinical Features

While classic pityriasis rosea is a quick clinical diagnosis, the less typical cases pose great difficulties. In about 50% of patients, the initial lesion is a singular sharply bordered red macule or papule on the nape or trunk. This lesion gradually expands over days creating a oval salmon plaque 2–10 cm in diameter, known as the herald patch (Fig. 43). The herald patch has a slightly sunken center with fine branny (pityriasiform) scale while at the periphery the plaque is slightly raised and the scales fade off towards the center. The later feature is important as the scales in a patch of tinea corporis fade towards the periphery. This pattern of scaling is known as collarette scale. On occasion, more than one herald patch may be present.

About 7–14 days (range hours to three months) after the appearance of the herald patch, multiple oval 0.5–1.5 mm macules, papules and plaques develop on the trunk and proximal extremities (Fig. 44). They tend to follow the skin lines, so that on the back they often produce a Christmas tree pattern. The secondary lesions have the same macroscopic features as the herald patch – central pseudoatrophy with fine scale and a peripheral collarette scale.

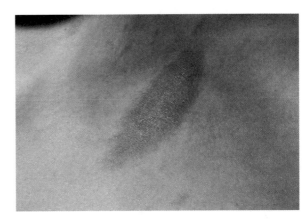

Fig. 43. Pityriasis rosea. Herald patch following the skin lines with erythema and fine scale.

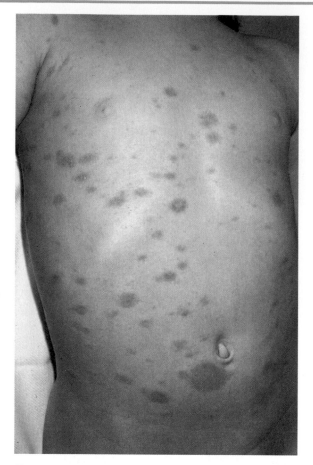

Fig. 44. Pityriasis rosea. Widespread distribution of oval salmon plaques following skin lines; lesion near umbilicus may be herald patch.

Smaller children often have atypical lesions, include hemorrhagic or lichenoid papules, vesicles, bullae and wheals. In such cases, the collarette scale is generally missing. Sometimes the disease is localized, involving a small area of the body, occasionally even unilateral. In other instances, the herald patch develops but then no diffuse rash follows. In pityriasis gigantea, all of the lesions achieve the size of a herald patch. In the even more extreme form, pityriasis marginata et circinata, these large patches become confluent.

The most puzzling variant is inverse pityriasis rosea. This is seen mainly in dark-skinned individuals and is so different from the ordinary disease that the diagnosis is a challenge. The lesions are papular, often annular, and favor the face, nape and distal extremities. In these individuals, the post-inflammatory hypopigmentation may be dramatic.

In rare instances, the oral mucosa is involved. Most such patients also have dramatic skin disease. Erythematous macules and patches, punctate hemorrhages, vesicles and small ulcers may be seen. The changes are similar to other viral enanthems, supporting the likely viral etiology of pityriasis rosea.

Finally, the course of the disease is unpredictable. Patients may continue to develop new lesions for several weeks. Sometimes as the first crop appears to be resolving, another flare will occur. While the average patient clears in about 4 weeks, it is wiser to tell the patient and parents that the usual course is 8–12 weeks, to avoid repeated worried consultations. Both post-inflammatory hypo- and hyperpigmentation may be seen. While most individuals only experience pityriasis rosea once, some individuals have the disease several times.

Symptoms

In most instances, pityriasis rosea is asymptomatic, but the patient or parents are upset by the dramatic appearance of the skin changes. About 25% of the patients complain of pruritus; this number is higher in inverse pityriasis rosea. About 5% have other signs of a possible viral infection including headache, gastrointestinal complaints, fever, arthralgias, and malaise.

Diagnosis

The diagnosis can usually be made clinically. If the case is atypical, it will probably be diagnosed incorrectly, as there are no confirmatory laboratory tests and the histopathology is not distinctive.

Table 39. Differential diagnosis of pityriasis rosea

Diagnosis	Distinguishing Features
■ **Tinea corporis**	Plaque with central clearing, advancing scale; fewer lesions; does not follow skin lines; in children, usually animal contact; KOH and culture positive
■ **Secondary syphilis**	Often history of primary lesion; fever, lymphadenopathy; involvement of palms and soles; more monotonous exanthem with red-brown tones; positive syphilis serology (mandatory in pregnancy; never wrong to order)
■ **Guttate psoriasis**	Often follows streptococcal pharyngitis; uniform silvery scales; scalp and face involvement; does not follow skin lines; positive Auspitz sign
■ **Nummular dermatitis**	Round lesion with papulo-vesicles, later scales and crusts; distal extremities; ± associated with atopic dermatitis; does not follow skin lines
■ **Lichen planus**	Violaceous flat-topped papules; pruritic; common around wrists; Wickham striae; does not follow skin lines
■ **Seborrheic dermatitis**	Irregular erythematous patches around hair line, naso-labial fold, behind ears; occasionally on trunk (petaloid seborrheic dermatitis); does not follow skin lines
■ **Viral exanthems**	Usually not scaly; does not follow skin lines; often fever, lymphadenopathy; viral serologic testing available
■ **Drug eruption**	History of medication use; otherwise, can be identical
■ **Pityriasis lichenoides et varioliformis acuta**	Usually hemorrhagic; never has herald patch; does not follow skin lines

Differential Diagnosis

Pityriasis rosea is often described as a chameleon, for it can mimic so many different diseases, as shown in Table 39. The most important point is that pityriasis rosea and some exanthems of secondary syphilis are clinically identical, so that in case of clinical questions or pregnancy, syphilis serology is mandatory. Quite often, the herald patch is misdiagnosed as a patch of tinea corporis, so one should be extremely suspicious of pityriasis rosea when the history is that of a rapidly spreading fungal disease under treatment.

Therapy

Pityriasis rosea usually requires no treatment other than reassurance. The affected skin dries out easily and can then become pruritic; thus good skin care with a bland emollient cream is wise. Similarly, one cannot wash pityriasis rosea away, so bathing or showering should be restricted to cleaning dirty areas and followed by lubrication. Bath oils containing polidocanol maybe useful for reducing this aspect of the pruritus.

If the lesions are pruritic, we usually choose mid-potency topical corticosteroids (Table 40). They are applied once daily in the evening and combined with frequent lubrication, perhaps with the vehicle base. Some individuals find relief with a zinc oxide shake lotion; others find this too drying, in which case olive oil can be added to the mixture. Another possibility is an emollient cream or lotion with 5% polidocanol.

One can also prescribe oral antihistamines, especially at night. We usually chose dimethindene maleate or doxylamine succinate.

If the oral lesions are troublesome, triamcinolone acetonide in an oral adhesive base (for example, Kenalog in Orabase®) may be helpful, although some patients tolerate a corticosteroid gel not specifically designed for mucosa even better.

In widespread disease, and especially in inverse pityriasis rosea, the pruritus may be

Pityriasis Rosea

Table 40. Treatment of pityriasis rosea

Clinical Constellation	Treatment
■ **Asymptomatic**	No treatment needed; good skin care
■ **Few pruritic lesions**	Topical corticosteroids in the evening and emollients
■ **Multiple pruritic lesions**	Topical corticosteroids in the evening and emollients; emollient cream or lotion with 5% polidocanol; systemic antihistamines
■ **Severe generalized pruritus**	Short course of systemic corticosteroids (methylprednisolone 0.5 mg/kg daily for 3 days; then 0.25 mg/kg daily for 3 days; systemic antihistamines

so troublesome that a short burst of systemic corticosteroids is justified. We give methylprednisolone 0.5 mg/kg daily for 3 days and then 0.25 mg/kg daily for another 3 days. The relief is usually dramatic and rebound flares uncommon.

Oral antibiotics may also have a role in pityriasis rosea. In one study, patients with elevated acute phase proteins and a history of an antecedent upper airway infection (a small part of the entire pityriasis rosea spectrum in our practice) were treated with erythromycin 25–40 mg/kg daily in 4 divided doses for 14 days. More patients in the treated group than the control group cleared over 6 weeks, but the applicability and efficacy of this new approach requires confirmation. While UV phototherapy has long been employed for pityriasis rosea, we do not use it as the disease usually resolves spontaneously over a reasonable period of time.

References

Allen R.A., Janniger C.K., Schwartz R.A.: Pityriasis rosea. Cutis 56:198–202 (1995)

Arndt K.A., Paul B.S., Stern R.S., Parrish J.A.: Treatment of pityriasis rosea with UV radiation. Archives of Dermatology 119:381–382 (1983)

Björnberg A., Hellgren L.: Pityriasis rosea. A statistical, clinical and laboratory investigation of 826 patients and matched healthy controls. Acta Dermato-Venereologica 42 (Suppl 50):1–68 (1962)

Chuh A.A., Chiu S.S., Peiris J.S.: Human herpesvirus 6 and 7 in peripheral blood leucocytes and plasma in patients with pityriasis rosea by polymerase chain reaction: a prospective case control study. Acta Derm Venereol 81:289–290 (2001)

Drago F., Ranieri E., Malaguti F., Losi E., Rebora A.: Human herpesvirus 7 in pityriasis rosea. Lancet 349:1367–1368 (1997)

Karzon D.T., Hayner N.S., Winkelstein W. Jr., Barron A.L.: An epidemic of aseptic meningitis syndrome due to Echo virus type 6: a clinical study of Echo 6 infection. Pediatrics 29:418–431 (1962)

Leenutaphong V., Jiamton S.: UVB phototherapy for pityriasis rosea: a bilateral comparison study. Journal of the American Academy of Dermatology 33:996–999 (1995)

Leonforte J.F.: Pityriasis rosea: exacerbation with corticosteroid treatment. Dermatology 163:480–481 (1980)

Rubins S., Janniger C.K., Schwartz R.A.: Congenital and early acquired syphilis. Cutis 56:132–136 (1995)

Sherma P.K., Yadav T.P., Gautam R.K., Taneja N., Satyanarayana L.: Erythromycin in pityriasis rosea: a double blind, placebo-controlled clinical trial. Journal of the American Academy of Dermatology 42:241–244 (2000)

Watanabe T., Kawamura T., Jacob S.E., Aquilino E.A., Orenstein J.M., Black J.B., Blauvelt A.: Pityriasis rosea is associated with systemic active infection with both human herpesvirus-7 and human herpesvirus-6. J Invest Dermatol 119:793–797 (2002)

CHAPTER 18 Psoriasis

K. BROCKOW

Epidemiology

Psoriasis is one of the most common skin diseases with a prevalence of 1–2%. Childhood psoriasis is not uncommon. The average age of onset in children is 8 years; findings before two years are unexpected. About 25% of the individuals who eventually develop psoriasis manifest the disease before 15 years of age. In children, psoriasis is more common in girls. The family history is positive in about half the cases. Children in whom the disease starts early with initial involvement of the trunk and face tend to have a more severe form of the disease.

Pathogenesis

Even though the pathogenesis of psoriasis has been and remains the subject of intensive investigation, the final picture remains unclear. In the past, psoriasis was viewed as primarily an epidermal proliferative disease. Today, it is well accepted that the key event is a T cell dysregulation with a shift to a Th1 dominated inflammatory reaction. Genetic factors are also important. A large part of childhood-onset psoriasis patients have a positive family history. Streptococcal antigens are the best established trigger, although many other factors have been discussed. In adults, alcohol consumption and use of beta-blockers for arterial hypertension have to be considered as trigger factors.

Clinical Features

The classic lesion of untreated psoriasis is an erythematous plaque with thick silver-gray scale. The clinical spectrum of the disease is highly variable. Some patients have only a few plaques on the sites of predilection, such as the knees, elbows, lower back, scalp and retroauricular region (Fig. 45). Others have lesions covering their entire body. In such cases, the early lesions are small erythematous macules with thinner scale, which then enlarge, coalesce (Fig. 46) or even cover the entire skin (psoriatic erythroderma). Other clinical findings may include nail dystrophies, acral lesions, pustular lesions (both limited to the palms and soles, as well as widespread) and anogenital disease. The Köbner phenomenon is often seen in psoriasis; trauma or other forms of skin irritation lead to the induction of psoriasis in the affected areas. The course of psoriasis is chronic; in the case of spontaneous or therapy-induced remission, a relapse is to be expected.

In children, the most common type is guttate psoriasis, usually in association with a streptococcal pharyngitis. These patients typically have disseminated smaller sized plaques on face, trunk, and scalp. In small children psoriasis may present first in the anogenital area, often mistaken for napkin dermatitis. Other types of psoriasis are less common in the younger population.

The major systemic complication of psoriasis is psoriatic arthritis, a disabling, possibly mutilating psoriasis which may take

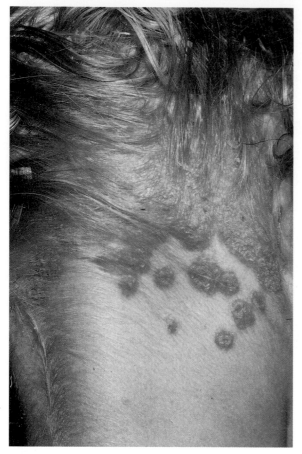

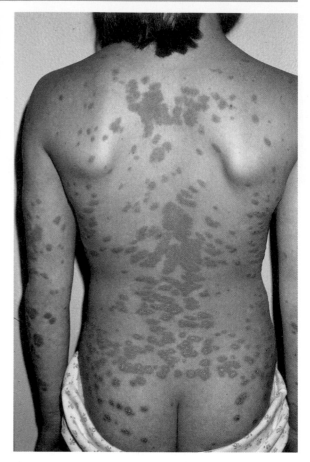

Fig. 45. Psoriasis. Erythematous coalesced plaques with transition to smaller, new lesions with silvery scales and also crusts.

Fig. 46. Psoriasis. Disseminated sharply bordered erythematous plaques on trunk and arms with areas of coalescence. Once again the smaller lesions more clearly show the classic silvery scales.

many forms. In childhood-onset psoriasis (type I), skin disease tends to be more severe and difficult to treat, but arthritis is more common in late-onset (type II) psoriasis.

Symptoms

While only 20–40% of psoriasis patients complain of pruritus, almost all suffer a marked impairment in the qualify of life, because of the "disfigurement" caused by the disease and the resulting social rejection.

Diagnosis

The diagnosis is usually made by the patient or the family. The answer is usually clinically obvious and a biopsy is rarely needed. One should always inquire about a family history. If psoriasis is suspected, it is wise to check the nails, scalp and gluteal cleft for typical but overlooked changes. When one peels the scale off a psoriasis lesion, one sees punctuate bleeding from the tortuous dermal capillaries; this is known as Auspitz sign.

Table 41. Differential diagnosis of psoriasis

Diagnosis	Distinguishing Features
■ **Lichen planus**	Flat-topped violaceous polygonal papules; no scale; pruritus; often mucosal involvement
■ **Pityriasis rosea**	Fine collarette scale; herald patch; follows skin lines, resolves spontaneously
■ **Seborrheic dermatitis**	Fine scale of scalp; eye brows, naso-labial fold, retroauricular area often involved
■ **Pityriasis lichenoides chronica**	Small erythematous papules on trunk with small compact scale (*Oblaten* scale)
■ **Pityriasis rubra pilaris**	Perifollicular erythema with keratotic papules; later coalescent papulo-squamous eruption with fine scale, salmon color and islands of sparing
■ **Secondary syphilis**	Disseminated small scaly papules; mucosal lesions; palms and soles involved; often hair loss; fever and lymphadenopathy; no pruritus; serology positive
■ **Tinea corporis**	Pruritic annular or nummular erythema with peripheral scale; KOH and culture positive

Differential Diagnosis

The major differential diagnostic considerations are shown in Table 41. The major considerations with multiple small lesions appearing acutely (i.e., guttate psoriasis) are pityriasis rosea, pityriasis lichenoides et varioliformis acuta and even secondary syphilis. When larger coin-shaped lesions are present, one may consider nummular dermatitis or tinea corporis. Pityriasis rubra pilaris is a puzzling papulo-squamous eruption which is considerably less common than psoriasis; often early involvement with the two diseases is hard to tell apart.

Therapy

Since a cure for psoriasis is not available, both the patient and the physician must direct their efforts towards avoiding or promptly treating flares of the disease. The major options are avoidance of possible triggers and intensive topical therapy, which is favored in children because it has few side effects. In difficult cases, either phototherapy or very rarely systemic therapy may be combined with aggressive topical therapy. Compliance is a problem in children. Many of the treatment regimens are time-consuming and messy. One must expend every effort to insure the cooperation of the child and parents.

In the case of guttate psoriasis, one should always exclude an acute infection with β-hemolytic streptococci, usually a pharyngitis. Appropriate tests include a throat culture, anti-streptolysin titer and urinalysis. If a streptococcal infection is identified, the child should be treated with oral penicillin (phenoxymethyl penicillin); the usual dosages are infants, 150,000 IU t.i.d.; age 1–6 years, 300,000 IU t.i.d.; >6 years, 500,000 IU t.i.d., in each case for 10 days. An alternative is erythromycin 30–50 mg/kg divided into 3–4 doses for 10 days. In cases with a clear history of febrile infection before the onset of skin disease, we tend to treat with oral antibiotics even if streptococcal infection cannot be proven by laboratory investigations.

If the child suffers from recurrent streptococcal pharyngitis and then flares of psoriasis, a tonsillectomy is worth considering. Although there is no large study supporting this approach, we have been impressed in a number of cases. Children with poor oral hygiene and multiple caries may also do better if this aspect of their health is improved.

One should also inquire what the parents and children suspect could be triggers. Possibilities include other infections or mechanical trauma (e.g., inadequate clothing or excessive combing in scalp disease). Finally, one should discuss the possibility of emotional triggers, such as family, school or social problems; only when these are brought into the open can they possibly be addressed.

Topical Therapy

Treating psoriasis means spending a great deal of time taking care of one's skin. Every physician prescribing complex treatment regimens should spend one weekend at home applying an ointment to 50% of their body q.i.d., taking medicated baths, and then applying other creams or ointment to various spots for varying lengths of time, removing them in specific ways. It is not easy!

In addition, the treatment must be adjusted to the extent of the disease. If one attempts to treat widespread disease with topical agents, one must at least prescribe large enough amounts that it is possible to treat the disease. For example, a 10 year old probably needs 15–30 g of a cream or ointment to cover their entire body. If one prescribes b.i.d. treatment to 25% of the body and gives a 30 g tube for two weeks, then something has to give – and it is compliance.

■ **Routine Skin Care.** It is important to convince the child with psoriasis that their skin requires care, even when they are doing well. Mechanical irritation or dryness can facilitate a flare of their disease, so the child should keep their skin lubricated with an economical emollient cream or ointment. In addition, bath soaks using a bath oil are very helpful.

■ **Removal of Scales.** A firm rule of psoriasis treatment is that every effort should be made to reduce the amount of scale so that the various medications can penetrate into the lesions better. We prefer 5% salicylic acid (range 3–10%) in an ointment base, applied to the lesions once or twice daily for 3 days (Table 42). If the scales are stubborn, overnight occlusion with a plastic kitchen wrap is effective. When salicylic acid is applied to wide areas in children, there is a

Table 42. Useful topical agents for childhood psoriasis

1. Keratolytics
   - ■ Scale-removing ointment
     Rx_
     salicylic acid 5.0 (3.0-10.0)
     ointment base ad 100.0

   - ■ Scale-removing oil
     Rx_
     salicylic acid 3.0
     olive oil ad 100.0

2. Anthralin
   - ■ Anthralin ointment
     Rx_
     anthralin 1/16 %–2.0%
     salicylic acid 3.0
     ointment base ad 100.0

   - ■ Short contact anthralin therapy
     Rx_
     anthralin 1/2%–2%
     salicylic acid 3.0
     ointment base ad 100.0

3. Modified Castellani solution
   Rx_
   chlorhexidine gluconate 5.0
   acetone 5.0
   fuchsin 4% in ethanol 10.0
   water ad 100.0

risk of salicylate poisoning, so that we start by only treating one side of the body. We do not use salicylic acid in children under 3 years of age.

An alternative is urea (5–12%) in an ointment base. Used in the same way, urea causes some stinging initially, but this is less of a problem when the product is applied to scaly skin than when it is used as a humectant on dry skin.

In addition, tub soaks with bath oils are helpful. We do not recommend salt solutions for bathing in children as they are often irritating and can cause corrosion of the drainage pipes.

■ **Anthralin.** One of the most effective and safest topical agents for psoriasis is anthralin. It has a cytostatic effect and produces marked inflammation; in German, there is a saying, "psoriasis disappears in the fire of anthralin". The response is prompter than with other agents and the remissions, longer lasting. On the other hand, considerable dermatologic experience is required to use the agent because of its irritant effects. We use a very detailed consent form and prefer to hospitalize the patients for several days at the start of therapy so they can be instructed in the use of anthralin.

One disadvantage of anthralin is that it discolors the skin (temporary) as well as the bedding and clothing (permanently). The patient and parents must be warned about this problem, but it is addressable. The anthralin must be applied exactly to the psoriasis lesions, and the patient should use old clothing and bedding. The anthralin is applied at night in the traditional regimens and then washed off in the morning using a syndet. The skin can be re-lubricated with a bath oil or emollient cream.

The trick with anthralin is to obtain a mild inflammation of the skin, but not a irritant toxic dermatitis. If the later occurs, the anthralin is stopped for 1–3 days and a midpotency corticosteroid is used. To avoid this, we start with a 1/64% or 1/32% anthralin (depending on the child's age), 3% salicylic acid in a water-in-oil ointment (Table 42). The salicylic acid is not only a keratolytic but also a preservative for anthralin. After 3–4 days, the concentration of the anthralin is doubled. The process continues until a 2% concentration is reached or healing has occurred. Some patients never advance past a ½–1% concentration. The face and flexural areas are more sensitive and are always treated with relatively lower concentrations.

One notices the effect of anthralin as the inflammation in the psoriatic plaques begins to resolve. At the end of treatment, the former plaques are often pale or white; this is known as psoriatic leukoderma. The patient must continue good basic skin care with regular lubrication of the skin.

Short contact anthralin therapy is more acceptable to many patients. Higher concentrations are used for a shorter time period.

Commercially available creams contain anthralin in increasing concentrations. One starts with the lowest concentration, applies it to the lesions, waits 5 minutes, and washes it off. The cream forms are especially handy because they are easy to remove, although they still stain. Every 3 days one increases the time by 5 minutes. When 30–45 minutes are reached, it is time to move up to the next concentration. This is obviously a time-consuming process, but most patients are happy to comply because the demands other than time are minimal and the remissions, once obtained, are lengthy.

■ **Vitamin D Analogs.** The topical vitamin D analogs stimulate the differentiation of keratinocytes and block their proliferation. Two quite similar agents are available around the world – calcipotriol and tacalcitol. Both are ideally suited to treating the early, not markedly infiltrated or heavily scaled, lesions of psoriasis. A third one, calcitriol, has been approved recently in various European countries. The greatest advantage of the vitamin D analogs is that they are user friendly; they are not messy, do not stain and do not have the "feared" corticosteroid side effects.

In adults, the recommended maximum dose of calcipotriol is <15 g/daily (divided in two applications) and less than 30% of body surface, respectively. For tacalcitol <10 g/daily (single application) and <15% of body surface are considered safe. Adhering to this maximum dose, systemic effects are not seen, although there is a possibility of hypercalcemia if they are overused. The maximum safe dose for children has not been determined. Tacalcitol is first approved at 12 years of age, while calcipotriol ointment is approved for 6 years of age. It is unclear if there are true differences in safety or just different marketing strategies. Both substances can cause burning and irritation, especially on the face and in the flexures. They should be used carefully in this areas. Vitamin D analogs should not be combined with salicylic acid or applied directly before UV irradiation, as both inactivate them.

Although some studies show that calcipotriol is superior to betamethasone valerate and anthralin, our personal experience is that they are weaker. In a well-designed study in children, calcipotriol was only slightly better than placebo (intensive skin care). We use the vitamin D analogs only in minimally infiltrated lesions, as often seen in acute flares and guttate psoriasis.

Calcitriol is the physiologic form of vitamin D3, also available as a topical agent. It has not been studied in children. The manufacturer's recommendation is not to treat more than 35% of the skin surface and <30 g/daily.

■ **Tars.** In the past, tars were used extensively either alone or with UV irradiation in the treatment of psoriasis. Today, they have been replaced by products that are cosmetically more elegant, as tars are messy and smell bad. In addition, there are concerns about their role as carcinogens; thus, we no longer employ them in the treatment of childhood psoriasis.

■ **Topical Corticosteroids.** In the USA, topical corticosteroids are the most commonly substance prescribed for psoriasis. The more potent products, especially under occlusion, work dramatically, but the downside is the tendency for a prompt rebound flare when the product is stopped and the well-known topical side effects (skin thinning, telangiectases). Thus, topical corticosteroids are restricted to small areas which are for anatomic reasons not very likely to show side effects, such as the scalp, nails, palms and soles. In addition, they may be useful to obtain a quick response on the face. The areas that are particularly likely to show corticosteroid side effects are the face (see Chapter 15, Perioral Dermatitis), axillae and anogenital region.

The newer corticosteroids with their dramatically improved risk-benefit ratio, such as mometasone furoate, methylprednisolone aceponate and prednicarbate, are extremely useful in children, but still should only be used for a short period of time and possibly in combination with other therapeutic regimens to obtain a sustained response.

■ **Phytotherapeutic Agents.** In Germany, there has been a dramatic revival of interest in phytopharmaceuticals. *Mahonia aquifolium* (Oregon grape [although not a grape] and state flower of Oregon) has been shown to have an anti-inflammatory, anti-psoriatic effect but in our experience it is minimal. We sometimes use it as a supplement to short contact anthralin therapy or in very young children with involvement of the anogenital area.

■ **Treatment of Specific Locations.** As one starts to treat psoriasis, one of the first things which becomes clear is that what works at one body site may not work at another.

■ **Scalp.** Here we like to use 3–10% salicylic acid in olive oil, almond oil, castor oil or in an ointment, which can be applied overnight under a shower cap. An alternative is a 10% urea cream or ointment used the same way. In the morning, the medication and the loosened scales are removed with a keratolytic shampoo. After a few days, the scalp is "debrided" enough that medications can be effectively applied. Since corticosteroid atrophy does not occur on the scalp, topical corticosteroids are the agent of choice. Either a gel or lotion can be applied once daily. Some patients may prefer a cream for smaller areas or if they have little hair. In severe cases, these can be used over night as well. After a few days, improvement is apparent and the frequency of application can be reduced. Vitamin D analogs can also be used on the scalp; they come as scalp solutions, which some people find very irritating due to their alcoholic base. The response is much slower than that to corticosteroids.

■ **Face.** The ear and external auditory canal are best treated with corticosteroid creams or ointments. A lotion appears logical, but patients often use it as ear drops without success, just causing occlusion. The face is very sensitive to corticosteroids; one should not use them for more than a few days and instead concentrate on repeated use of emollient creams.

■ **Intertriginous Areas.** Here we prefer to use an modified colorless Castellani solution (Table 42). An alternative in the future might be calcitriol as it is much less irritating than tacalcitol and calcipotriol, but at the time being there is no data on resorption and potential side effects in intertriginous areas.

■ **Phototherapy.** If topical therapy alone is not successful, one can combine either anthralin or vitamin D analog treatment with UV irradiation. Narrow band 311 nm (Phillips TL01) UVB treatment appears ideal for psoriasis. One should be very reluctant to use phototherapy in children. The life time risk of development of a malignant melanoma or squamous cell carcinoma is significantly increased in psoriatic patients receiving repeatedly phototherapy. For this same reason, we do not use PUVA therapy (psoralens + UVA) in children, even though it is extremely effective.

■ **Systemic Therapy**

Only in rare instances is systemic treatment needed in childhood psoriasis. Antibiotics may be helpful for guttate psoriasis. Systemic corticosteroids are not appropriate; the side effects and rebound risk are too significant. Methotrexate is only appropriate in severe psoriatic arthritis of childhood, a rare disorder. We are similarly reluctant to use other cytostatic agents or cyclosporine A. Oral retinoids (acitretin 0.5 mg/kg daily) are effective for pustular psoriasis and psoriatic erythroderma; there is enough experience with their use in children with disorders of keratinization so that the potential problems with the skeletal system (premature closure of the epiphyses) can be avoided by limiting use. Appropriate control investigations (especially CBC, liver enzymes, cholesterol and triglycerides, as well as documentation of growth) are mandatory.

References

Burden A.D.: Management of psoriasis in childhood. Clin Exp Dermatol 24:341–345 (1999)

Hurwitz S.: Clinical Pediatric Dermatology, pp. 105–117, 2nd ed. Saunders, Philadelphia (1993)

Lacour M., Mehta-Nikhar B., Atherton D.J., Harper J.I.: An appraisal of acitretin therapy in children with inherited disorders of keratinization. Br J Dermatol 134:1023–1029 (1996)

Nyfors A.: Psoriasis in children. Acta Dermato-Venereologica (Suppl) 95:47–53 (1981)

Oranje A.P., Marcoux D., Svensson A., Prendiville J., Krafchik B., Toole J., Rosenthal D., de Ward-van der Spek F.B., Molin L., Axelsen M.: Topical calcipotriol in childhood psoriasis. Journal of the American Academy of Dermatology 36:203–208 (1997)

Owen C.M., Chalmers R.J., O'Sullivan T., Griffiths C.E.: Antistreptococcal interventions for guttate and chronic plaque psoriasis. Cochrane Database Systematical Reviews 2000:CD001976

Simpson K.R., Lowe N.J.: Trends in topical psoriasis therapy. International Journal of Dermatology 33:333–336 (1994)

Zvulunov A., Anisfeld A., Metzker A.: Efficacy of short-contact therapy with dithranol in childhood psoriasis. International Journal of Dermatology 33:808–810 (1994)

CHAPTER 19 Scabies

O. BRANDT

Epidemiology

Scabies is a worldwide infectious disease whose incidence in Germany has increased in recent years. Sex, age, race, and socioeconomic status play only a small role in the epidemiology of scabies. The scabies mite is almost always transferred by direct body contact. Children and especially small children have a greater risk of infection than adults. Mothers of small children are more likely to acquire the infection than fathers. Those living under extremely confined circumstances, as well as immunosuppressed individuals, are also at greater risk.

Pathogenesis

The etiologic agent of scabies is the mite *Sarcoptes scabiei variatio hominis*, in the class Arachnida, order Acari, suborder Acaridida. The adult female mite has a dome-shaped body 0.3–0.4 mm long and can be spotted with the naked eye. The male is only half as large. As with all arachnids, *Sarcoptes scabiei* has four pairs of legs; the posterior pair have each a long hair.

Following mating, the male dies while the female seeks a suitable spot on the host into which to burrow. Using her strong mandible, she tunnels into the deeper layers of the stratum corneum and then advances 0.5–5.0 mm daily, depositing two to three eggs in the tunnel each day. The six-legged larva hatch after 3–7 days and then develop through a nymph stage into eight-legged adults. An adult female can live for up to two months. On average an infected individual has 10–15 mites on their body. Infants and immunosuppressed individuals may have many more mites, while in crusted or Norwegian scabies, the number is enormous.

The pruritus which results from an scabies infestation is a Type IV delayed hypersensitivity reaction. This means that upon initial exposure to *Sarcoptes scabiei*, no one itches. It takes at least a few weeks, usually 2–6, before an immune response to mite saliva, feces or other antigens develops. Then the pruritus starts. Upon re-exposure, the individual starts to itch within a few hours. The mite can, thus, be easily transferred before the carrier has either pruritus or skin lesions.

It is also possible for a human to become infested by mites from an animal, usually a dog. There is marked species specificity, so that a dog mite cannot reproduce on a human. Thus, mite infections with non-human arthropods are always self-limited, although they may be very pruritic.

Clinical Features

In older children, adolescents and adults, the hallmark of scabies is intense pruritus, worse at night, associated with excoriations (Fig. 47) and pruritic tiny papules on the hands and feet, intertriginous areas, umbilicus, belt line and anogenital region. Places which are particularly likely to be involved are the interdigital spaces, the volar aspect of the wrist, palms and soles (Fig. 48). Scaly

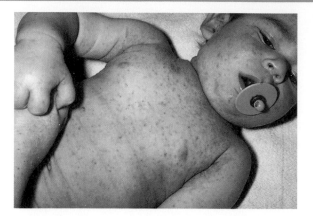

Fig. 47. Scabies. Disseminated papules and excoriations, as well as flexural dermatitic changes.

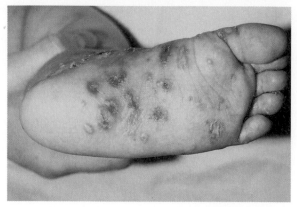

Fig. 49. Scabies. Papules, pustules, crusts and excoriations on sole.

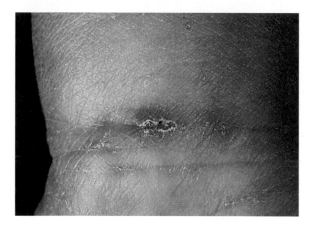

Fig. 48. Scabies. Excoriated papule in typical volar location.

macules on the nipple or glans penis are highly suggestive of scabies. If one looks closely, sometimes tunnels with a tiny dark point (the female) at the end can be found. In other instances, one only sees excoriations.

While the face and scalp are spared in older patients, these regions are often involved in infants and small children and must be treated. In addition, the lesions are more likely to be vesicular or pustular. Typical sites are the hands, feet, and gluteal cleft (Fig. 49). The excoriations are once again prominent and it can be extremely difficult to find intact tunnels and to identify the mite with certainty.

Secondary infections of the excoriations with *Staphylococcus aureus* or *Streptococcus*

pyogenes may occur, causing impetigo. One should be alert to potential complications of the bacterial infections such as staphylococcal scalded skin syndrome or acute glomerulonephritis. In order to avoid such problems, if secondary infection is identified, the patient should be treated with the appropriate antibiotics.

An uncommon variant of scabies is crusted or Norwegian scabies. Such patients have massive crusts which consist primarily of scabies mites, so that they have millions of mites on their body. Often the infestation is overlooked as psoriasis or a crusted dermatitis. Obviously such individuals are extremely contagious. Crusted scabies is seen today most often in HIV/AIDS, but is also a problem in Down syndrome patients and other immunosuppressed individuals. A single patient with crusted scabies in a nursing home or child care center can infest many other patients, workers, and visitors.

The exact opposite is scabies of the cleanly. In individuals who frequently and carefully wash their skin (or have it washed in the case of infants and small children), it can be extremely difficult to find a mite. The patients complain of pruritus and have excoriations, but little else. In patients being treated with systemic or topical corticosteroids, sometimes the pruritus may be suppressed as the mites flourish (scabies incognita). Such patients are also highly infective.

After scabies has been treated, nodules may persist for weeks to months. They are most common in infants and children and typically seen in the anogenital or axillary regions. Microscopically they contain a dense lymphocytic infiltrate, so that they are usually diagnosed as a pseudolymphoma.

Symptoms

The cardinal symptom is intense pruritus, worse at night. Children may suffer from sleep deprivation and thus be irritable or upset during the day. Some infants are so miserable that they fail to eat and drink properly, so that scabies can even become life-threatening. Once the infestation has been treated, the pruritus does not disappear immediately but may last for 3–7 days.

Diagnosis

Although scabies should be suspected in any case of unexplained pruritus, especially if worse at night or present in multiple family members, there are many causes of itching and the diagnosis can only be made with certainty when *Sarcoptes scabiei*, its eggs or feces are identified.

The best place to find the mite is at the end of a tunnel. The tunnels are slightly elevated, often a few mm long and have a dark spot at their end; this is the female. While she can normally be seen with the naked eye, there are also tricks. If fountain pen ink is dripped onto a suspected area, allowed to sit for a few seconds and then wiped off, some ink may remain in a tunnel. Dermatoscopy is another way to identify a female. A drop of examining fluid is placed on the skin and then the dermatoscope is used to search for tunnels; the female at the end often resembles a hang glider. One must be certain to carefully disinfect the dermatoscope.

Once a suspicious site has been identified, a drop of mineral oil is placed on the skin and the tiny bump popped or scarified with a medium caliber injection needle. The female, eggs or feces tend to cling to the needle and can be transferred to a glass slide for microscopic study.

Differential Diagnosis

The differential diagnostic considerations are shown in Table 43. While there are many other pruritic skin diseases, they usually offer other clues. When pustular lesions are seen on the palms and soles, one must consider infantile acropustulosis and dyshidrotic dermatitis.

Therapy

It is often impossible to find a *Sarcoptes scabiei* and make the definite diagnosis of scabies. Thus, when there is a significant clinical suspicion (itching worse at night, multiple family members itching), a course of treatment for scabies is appropriate. As a rule, we never re-treat for scabies without finding the bug.

Not only the patient but all contact individuals must be treated. In most instances, this means treating the immediately family, although in some instances one is confronted with treating an entire kindergarten or day care center. Here a bit of caution and common sense is needed. Finally, in older children, adolescents and adults, treatment from the neck downwards with a standard scabicide is usually adequate, but in infants, the therapeutic approach becomes more troublesome. Here treatment must cover the entire body, including the face and scalp, although one must avoid the perioral and periorbital regions to avoid mucosal irritation. In addition, not all scabicides are safe in infancy, complicating the picture further.

Table 43. Differential diagnosis of scabies

Diagnosis	Distinguishing Features
■ **Atopic dermatitis**	Patches of dermatitis, usually flexural; papules uncommon; diaper area usually spared; pruritus may be just as intense
■ **Seborrheic dermatitis**	Pruritus mild; usually in infants with thick greasy scales; rare in older children
■ **Contact dermatitis**	Uncommon in children; sharply localized
■ **Arthropod bite reaction**	Papular lesions often with central punctum; appear suddenly and synchronously
Pustular acral lesions	
■ **Infantile acropustulosis**	No lesions elsewhere; can be present at birth; family members not involved
■ **Dyshidrotic dermatitis**	Rare in infants; tense clear 1–3 mm vesicles

Table 44. Treatment of scabies

Agent	Dosage Regimen
■ **Permethrin**	Single overnight application, washing in a.m.
■ **Lindane**	Overnight application on three consecutive days; in small children, four treatments (one half of body each time); washing in a.m.
■ **Benzyl benzoate**	Applied twice daily for three days, washing in a.m. of fourth day

Topical Therapy

■ **Permethrin.** Permethrin is the standard agent of choice for scabies worldwide. In most countries, it is available as a 5% cream. A single application is effective in over 90% of patients (Table 44). In Germany, the product must be compounded, so that we use a 2.5% cream for children less than five years of age.

The cream is applied at night and washed off in the morning with soap and water. In newborns, the cream is washed off after 6 hours. If the palms and soles are affected, the treatment should be repeated in 10 days, as the thick stratum corneum in these regions offers the mite excellent protection.

Permethrin is not at all irritating. In rare cases a patient may complain of burning or erythema. A problem with all scabies treatments is that patients tend to overuse the product, figuring if one treatment is good, five are better. Thus, the usual toxicological rules loose some of their relevance. In the case of permethrin, it is so non-toxic with less than 2% absorption that even with repeated misuse, toxicity is not a problem. Permethrin is widely used in pregnant and nursing women, as well as in infants. Permethrin is not approved for infants below 2 years of age, but this is probably the best choice if therapy is needed in this age group. Very small children should be treated one body half after the other on consecutive days. Since lindane is neurotoxic, many physicians do not use it in patients with neurological disease, preferring the non-toxic permethrin.

■ **Lindane (gamma benzene hexachloride).** Lindane was for years the standard scabicide worldwide. It too is applied in the evening and washed off the next morning. Consensus has never been reached on the best application plan. In Germany, lindane (0.3%, Jacutin®) is applied for three consecutive evenings; in the USA most commercially available products contain 1% lindane and most treat twice, one week apart, while others endorse a single application, which is our usual approach. In two smaller trials, lindane appeared less effective than permethrin, but in the largest trial they were comparable in effectiveness. Resistance is occasionally observed.

The main problems with lindane are that it is better absorbed and neurotoxic. Patients may describe headache, dizziness or nausea after applying lindane. In addition, in cases of extreme overuse, elevated serum levels are occasionally documented and, in rare cases, permanent neurological damage.

For these reasons we observe the following precautions:

■ In the US lindane is not used in children under three years of age; in some European countries it is used under the age of three in a hospital setting, where one body half is treated on days 1 and 3, the other body half on days 2 and 4.
■ It is not used in pregnant or nursing women.
■ Patients with an abnormal epidermal barrier (atopic dermatitis, other widespread skin diseases) or reduced subcutaneous fat are also not treated.
■ Lindane penetrates moist skin much better than dry, so it should not be applied after bathing or showering.
■ Lindane is very irritating, so that the pruritus may increase despite successful elimination of mites. The use of emollients or even low- to mid-potency steroids after the three day treatment regimen is helpful.

■ **Benzyl Benzoate.** This agent is more popular in developing lands as an inexpensive scabicide and pediculicide. Benzyl benzoate is derived from balsam of Peru or synthesized synthetically. It is available in Germany in both a 10% and 25% concentration. It is applied b.i.d. for 3 days without bathing or showering and removed on the fourth day by washing. The product is intrinsically irritating and the repeated applications do not help. In addition, allergic contact dermatitis may develop, presumably because of the connections to balsam of Peru.

■ **Crotamiton.** This product is sold as a scabicide but is not very effective. It does have an anti-pruritic action which makes it attractive to some prescribers, as does its superb safety

profile. It is the only scabicide approved for use in newborns, as well as pregnant and nursing women. In order to achieve even a modest efficacy, crotamiton must be applied daily for five consecutive days.

■ Systemic Therapy

The systemic treatment of scabies is accomplished using ivermectin, a macrolide agent initially employed against worms by veterinarians and now used for onchocerciasis. A single oral dose of 200 µg/kg cures over 80% of patients. Ivermectin can be used safely and effectively in older children. It lends itself to treating large populations at risk, such as nursing homes, kindergartens or day care centers.

Ivermectin is not recommended for children under five years of age or those weighing less than 30 kg because of the risk of CNS side effects. In addition, it is not used in pregnant or nursing women.

■ Other Therapeutic Issues

■ **Crusted Scabies.** Today ivermectin is widely employed for crusted scabies, especially in HIV/AIDS. If one attempts to treat the disease with topical agents alone, then it is essential to somehow remove the crusts, using keratolytic agents such as salicylic acid ointments (see Chap. 8), prior to scabicides. In addition, the scalp and face must be treated, and multiple courses of therapy are required.

■ **Other Problems.** The pruritus should be treated with a systemic antihistamine until it relents. We prefer dimethindene maleate, doxylamine succinate or hydroxyzine. Secondary dermatitic changes also contribute to the pruritus, so that topical corticosteroids may also be useful. After several days of anti-inflammatory treatment, the scabies regimen will be less irritating.

The fingernails should be cut short so they produce less damage when used for scratching. In addition, any debris under the nails should be removed regularly, as the mites can be transferred through this site.

If there is a bacterial secondary infection, it should be treated. For streptococci, penicillin is usually chosen, while for staphylococci, a penicillinase-resistant penicillin is needed. First generation cephalosporins are effective against both bacteria (Chapter 9).

Once the treatment is completed, the skin requires additional tender loving care. Careful attention should be paid to restoring the barrier function, using bath oils and emollient creams. If irritation or pruritus continues to be a problem, corticosteroids can be used for a few nights afterwards.

The persistent infiltrated nodules may cause problems for months. They can be treated with a higher potency topical steroid b.i.d.

■ **Supportive Measures.** The clothing and bedding should be washed. Items which cannot be washed can be dry clean or hung outdoors for 48 hours, or indoors for 1 week in a place where human contact is impossible (an attic or garage for example). Upholstery, carpets and rugs should be vacuumed. Only rarely is chemical treatment needed, as for example when an infected individual has slept on a sofa.

All contact individuals should be examined and/or treated. This is easy to write but hard to do. In some instances, such as when the father is working but has marked pruritus, he can be treated without be examined. On the other hand, if 50 children are in a kindergarten, one must be more selective.

If animal scabies is suspected, the pets in question as carriers should be examined by a veterinarian who is informed of the problem. This issue is far more common than usually suspected. One study showed that in 50% of cases when a pet owner had pruritus, there was a connection with their pets.

References

Burkhart C.N., Burkhart C.G.: Before using ivermectin therapy for scabies. Pediatric Dermatology 19:478–479 (1999)

Fölster-Holst R., Rufli T., Christophers E.: Die Skabiestherapie unter besonderer Berücksichtigung des frühen Kindesalters, der Schwangerschaft und Stillzeit. Hautarzt 51:7–13 (2000)

Meinking T.L., Taplin D.: Infestations. In: Schachner L.A., Hansen R.C. (eds.) Pediatric Dermatology, 2nd ed., pp. 1367–1381. Churchill Livingstone, New York (1995)

Molinaro M., Schwartz R., Janniger C.K.: Scabies. Cutis 56:317–321 (1995)

Orkin M., Maibach H.: Scabies treatment: current considerations. Current Problems in Dermatology 24:151–156 (1996)

Purvis R.S., Tyring S.K.: An outbreak on lindane-resistant scabies treated with permethrin 5% cream. J Am Acad Dermatol 25:1015–1016 (1991)

Quaterman M.J., Lesher J.L.: Neonatal scabies treated with permethrin 5% cream. Pediatr Dermatol 11:264–266 (1994)

Usha V., Gopalakrishnan Nair T.V.: A comparative study of oral ivermectin and topical permethrin cream in the treatment of scabies. Journal of the American Academy of Dermatology 236–240 (2000)

Walker G.J.A, Johnstone P.W.: Interventions for treating scabies. In: The Cochrane Library, Issue 4. Oxford: Update Software (2002)

CHAPTER 20 Seborrheic Dermatitis

T. SCHMIDT

Epidemiology

Infantile seborrheic dermatitis is most common during the first three months of life, with a range of 2–12 weeks. Occasionally the disease appears as late as 1½ years of age. Although both an association with atopic dermatitis and psoriasis and an increased frequency within families have been discussed, a pattern of inheritance has not been clearly shown. In our opinion, infantile seborrheic dermatitis is a specific disease entity which has a good prognosis as it almost always resolves spontaneously within 6–8 weeks. Except for the diaper area, recurrences are uncommon. While atopic dermatitis has become much more common in recent years, infantile seborrheic dermatitis has dropped in frequency.

Pathogenesis

The pathogenesis of infantile seborrheic dermatitis remains unclear. A number of possible contributing factors have been identified including increased production of sebum because of elevated maternal hormones or increased adrenocorticosteroid production in infancy as well as distorted fatty acid metabolism because of an inadequate output of δ6-desaturase. Colonization with *Malassezia furfur (Pityrosporum ovale, Pityrosporum orbiculare)* has also been considered relevant, but recent studies have failed to confirm this association.

Clinical Features

The two sites which are most commonly involved are the scalp and diaper region (Fig. 50). On the scalp the area most commonly affected is the temporal region which is covered by a thick micaceous scale, known in American slang as cradle cap (Fig. 51). The scale truly may resemble a cap, sitting on a surprisingly non-inflamed background, but thick, firmly adherent, yellowish and with small splits and tears. The scalp disease may be the only sign of infantile seborrheic dermatitis. Even with extensive involvement, there is no risk of permanent alopecia and resolution is spontaneous.

When the rest of the body is affected, one usually sees somewhat finer scale and crust on erythematous patches and plaques. The pattern can be nummular, annular or polycyclic. In the intertriginous areas, there may be weeping lesions as well as painful fissures. There may also be scattered lesions on the trunk which can, on occasion, coalesce (Fig. 52).

An extreme variant of infantile seborrheic dermatitis is known as Leiner disease (erythrodermia desquamativa). Such infants have erythroderma with systemic signs and symptoms (failure to thrive, fever, anemia, vomiting, diarrhea, lymphadenopathy). The disease is extremely rare and the exact etiology is unclear; perhaps many factors combine to produce the dramatic clinical picture. The best established abnormalities are abnormal neutrophil chemotaxis and complement abnormalities. In any event, the pa-

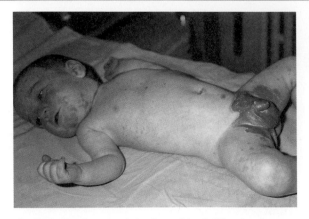

Fig. 50. Infantile seborrheic dermatitis. Striking involvement of diaper area with deep erythema and moist scales; milder erythema and scale affected the face and scalp.

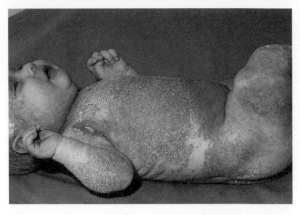

Fig. 52. Infantile seborrheic dermatitis. Disseminated disease with erythema and moist large scales involving the face and diaper area.

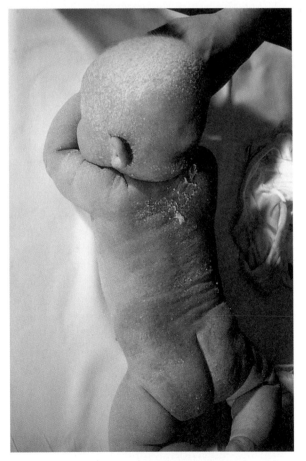

Fig. 51. Infantile seborrheic dermatitis. Thickened mica-like scale on scalp.

tients tend to experience bacterial and fungal superinfections which can lead to their demise.

Symptoms

Even with very prominent and widespread involvement, infantile seborrheic dermatitis is almost always asymptomatic. Occasionally the infant may scratch the lesions.

Diagnosis

The diagnosis can be made clinically and further investigations are not needed.

Differential Diagnosis

The most important differential diagnostic considerations are shown in Table 45.

Therapy

The main therapeutic possibilities are summarized in Table 46. In every instance one should keep in mind that spontaneous resolution is the rule and not be overaggressive.

Table 45. Differential diagnosis of infantile seborrheic dermatitis

Diagnosis	Distinguishing Features
■ **Atopic dermatitis**	Usually later onset (8–12 weeks); more pruritic; positive family history; more facial involvement and sparing of diaper area
■ **Psoriasis**	Uncommon in this age group; silvery scale; sometimes Auspitz sign positive
■ **Scabies**	Marked pruritus; other family members also itching; papules and papulo-vesicles, rather than thick scale; mites can be identified
■ **Nummular dermatitis**	Diaper area spared; dry coin-shaped lesions on trunk; usually yellow scales and crusts, as well as scattered serous papules
■ **Tinea corporis**	Uncommon in infants; diaper area spared; annular lesions with advancing border and central clearing; KOH and culture positive

■ Topical Therapy

■ **General Measures.** If the diaper area is involved, the mother should be encouraged to let the child go without diapers as much as is feasible and to employ non-occlusive diapers. The skin should be cleaned only when dirty with a mild neutral or acid syndet. Daily bathing in lukewarm water, using either a bath oil or perhaps an oatmeal bath (Aveeno® or Oilated Aveeno®), is also helpful.

■ **Scalp.** The scalp can be treated with olive or almond oil. We prefer to apply the oil at night, and wash the scalp in the morning. If the scales are stubborn, an ointment can be used in place of the oil; this is messier and requires more aggressive washing. Adding 3% salicylic acid to the oil makes the treatment more effective. Sometimes we cover the greased up scales with moist compresses or a moist cap for 3-5 hours before bathing the child, facilitating the descaling. If the disease is extensive, the moist compresses can cause overcooling. Once the scales have been removed, the underlying scalp can be treated with either a low-potency corticosteroid cream or an imidazole cream (using the latter for its anti-inflammatory as well as its anti-fungal properties). Another very effective step is the use of an imidazole shampoo, usually 2% ketoconazole shampoo, twice weekly for 2–4 weeks, and then later once weekly.

■ **Body.** On the body we prefer to use imidazole creams rather than corticosteroid creams, because of the better risk-benefit ratio. While we usually employ either clotrimazole or ketoconazole cream, there is no reason to think the other agents are not also effective. Usually a b.i.d. application suffices. If the imidazoles fail to help, one can use a low-potency corticosteroid cream once daily in the evening for 5–10 days in addition to the imidazole.

■ **Intertriginous Area.** In this difficult area we prefer a specific product – an elegant clotrimazole cream paste (Imazol Paste®) applied b.i.d. If lesions are weeping, they can be painted b.i.d. with an 0.1% aqueous gentian violet solution.

■ **Phytopharmaceuticals.** Borage seed oil is a plant oil containing 24% γ-linolenic acid. In our experience, as well as in the literature, the application of 0.5 mL of borage seed oil b.i.d. to the diaper area is an effective approach. Usually complete healing of not just the diaper area but also of scattered, non-treated lesions occurs in 10–12 days. Since recurrences are possible, we recommend applying the oil 2–3 times weekly until the child is 6 or 7 months old. Currently this is our treatment of choice, as it is cheap, safe, and effective.

■ Systemic Therapy

If pruritus appears to be severe, a sedating antihistamine (dimethindene maleate or doxylamine succinate) can be prescribed for a few nights until the topical regimen can take effect. Systemic antibiotics should be used for documented, severe secondary bacterial infec-

Table 46. Treatment of infantile seborrheic dermatitis

■ **General Recommendations**	Exposure	Fresh air
	Diapers	Non-occlusive
	Clothing	Light, airy; no wool or synthetic fabrics
	Cleansing	Neutral or acid syndet
	Shampooing	Mild shampoo
	Baths	Oatmeal or oil
■ **Topical Therapy** – Scalp	Loosening scale	Apply oil or ointment overnight; if severe, combine with wet compresses
	Anti-inflammatory	Low-potency corticosteroids
	Anti-inflammatory & anti-mycotic	Imidazole creams b.i.d. Imidazole shampoo 2× weekly, later less often
– Body	Anti-inflammatory	Low-potency corticosteroids
	Anti-inflammatory & anti-mycotic	Imidazole creams
– Intertriginous area	Anti-inflammatory & anti-mycotic	Imazol Paste® b.i.d. 0.1% aqueous gentian violet solution b.i.d.
■ **Phytopharmaceuticals**		Borage seed oil 0.5 mL to diaper area b.i.d.; after 10–12 days, switch to maintenance regimen 2–3× weekly
■ **Systemic Therapy**	Antihistamines	Sedating agent at bedtime (dimethindene maleate or doxylamine succinate)
	Antifungal agents	Only for gastrointestinal candidiasis
	Antibiotics	For culture-proven bacterial superinfections
	Corticosteroids	Methylprednisolone 1.0 mg/kg daily for severe disease (Leiner disease)

tions, while systemic antifungal agents are only indicated for proven oropharyngeal or gastrointestinal candidiasis. Systemic corticosteroids are almost never needed, except perhaps in the case of Leiner disease.

References

Menni S., Piccinno R., Baietta S., Ciuffreda A., Scotti L.: Infantile seborrhoeic dermatitis: seven-year follow-up and some prognostic criteria. Pediatric Dermatology 61:13–15 (1989)

Mimouni K., Mukamel M., Zeharia A., Mimouni M.: Prognosis of infantile seborrhoeic dermatitis. The Journal of Pediatrics 127:744–746 (1995)

Peter R.U., Richarz-Barthauer U.: Successful treatment and prophylaxis of scalp seborrhoeic dermatitis and dandruff with 2% ketoconazole shampoo: results of a multicentre, double-blind, placebo-controlled trial. British Journal of Dermatology 132:441–445 (1995)

Riuz-Maldonado R., Lopez-Martinez R., Perez Chavarria E.I., Castranon L.R., Tamayo L.: *Pityrosporum ovale* in infantile seborrhoeic dermatitis. Pediatric Dermatology 6:16–20 (1989)

Tollesson A., Frithz A., Stenlund K.: *Malassezia furfur* in infantile seborrhoeic dermatitis. Pediatric Dermatology 14:423–425 (1997)

Tolleson A., Graz A.: Borage oil, an effective new treatment for infantile seborrhoeic dermatitis. British Journal of Dermatology 129:5 (1993)

Wright M.C., Hevert F., Rosman T.: In vitro comparison of antifungal effects of a coal tar gel and a ketoconazole gel on *Malassezia furfur*. Mycoses 36:207–210 (1993)

Yates V.M., Kerr R.E.I., MacKie R.M.: Early diagnosis of infantile seborrhoeic dermatitis and atopic dermatitis-clinical features. British Journal of Dermatology 108:633–638 (1983)

Tinea Capitis

D. ABECK

Epidemiology

Tinea capitis occurs primarily in children with a peak incidence between 5–8 years of age.

Pathogenesis

Tinea capitis is a dermatophyte infection of the scalp. The most common cause in Europe is *Microsporum canis,* accounting for 50% of the cases. Most infections are transmitted from cats, not dogs, and often the story is that the child played with a cat while on vacation in southern Europe. Other causative dermatophytes include *Trichophyton verrucosum, Trichophyton violaceum, Trichophyton mentagrophytes*, and *Trichophyton rubrum*. In other parts of the world the most common cause is *Trichophyton tonsurans*. Infectious human tinea capitis, caused by *Microsporum audouinii,* caused epidemics in the post-World War II years but is rare today. The fungi elicit both an acute neutrophil-mediated inflammatory reaction and later a Type IV reaction.

Clinical Features

The typical clinical change is an expanding area of hair loss, with hairs broken off 2–3 mm above the skin surface. Scale may be prominent. In some instances there is little inflammation (Fig. 53), while in others there may more (Fig. 54). Sometimes there is neutrophilic inflammation about the hair follicles producing a red boggy mass which is secondarily infected and oozes pus; this disturbing change is known as a kerion (Fig. 55). In general, fungi transmitted from human to human such as *Trichophyton tonsurans* or *Microsporum audouinii* elicit less of an inflammatory response than those transferred from an animal to a child. In general, it is impossible to identify the causative dermatophyte by the clinical findings although *Trichophyton tonsurans* tends to produce little inflammation and broken off thickened hairs (because the fungi are within the hair shaft), producing a picture called "black dot" tinea.

Symptoms

In most instances tinea capitis is asymptomatic. More severe and deeper involvement may lead to pruritus. Children with kerion may have systemic signs and symptoms including fever, malaise, headache, nausea, vomiting, and lymphadenopathy.

Diagnosis

The diagnosis can be suspected clinically but should be confirmed. Wood light examination may help identify *Microsporum*, as infected hairs fluoresce yellow-green. A negative Wood light examination *does not* exclude a tinea capitis as *Trichophyton* do not fluoresce and even with *Microsporum* there may be negative findings.

The mainstays of diagnosis are the identification of the fungi with KOH examination

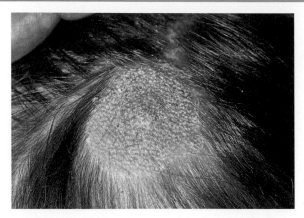

Fig. 53. Tinea capitis. Circular area of alopecia with fine scale and no evidence of inflammation. Causative agent: *Microsporum canis.*

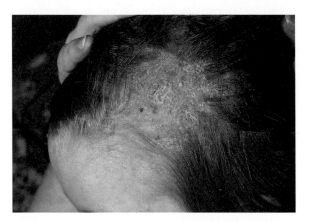

Fig. 54. Tinea capitis. Area of alopecia with erythema as well as yellow crusts and scales. Causative agent: *Microsporum canis.*

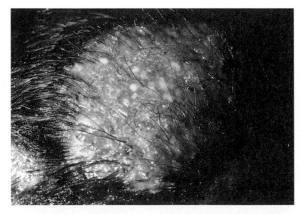

Fig. 55. Tinea capitis. Kerion with erythema, alopecia, boggy inflammation and pustules.

and fungal culture. Both plucked hairs and scale should be examined under the microscope, searching for fungal hyphae. The infected hairs are often easier to pluck than normal. The scalp should be cleaned with alcohol prior to taking the culture in order to avoid bacterial contamination. If pustules are present, their contents should be examined in the same way; in addition, a bacterial culture can be obtained. If the KOH examination is clearly positive, therapy can be started while waiting for the results of the culture which takes 1-3 weeks.

A common problem is that the scalp lesion has been previously treated with antiseptic, antibacterial or antifungal agents, making the positive diagnosis a challenge. Our approach in such cases when we cannot identify fungi with the KOH examination is to discontinue all treatment for a week and then re-assess the child. During the interval, an emollient cream can be applied to the lesion at night and then washed out in the morning. This approach will loosen scales, make the subsequent evaluation easier and retain the confidence of the parents. If there is marked crusting, wet soaks with compresses may speed the removal of scales.

Differential Diagnosis

The major differential diagnostic considerations are shown in Table 47. The most common challenges are trichotillomania, psoriasis, and atopic dermatitis.

Therapy

Tinea capitis always requires systemic treatment, accompanied by appropriate topical measures. The systemic antifungal agents eradicate the fungus while the topical approach is designed to more rapidly reduce the risk of transmission to others.

In Germany, only griseofulvin is officially approved for the treatment of tinea capitis. If one does choose to use griseofulvin, a dai-

Table 47. Differential diagnosis of tinea capitis

Diagnosis	Distinguishing Features
■ **Psoriasis**	Typical lesions elsewhere; rarely pustules on scalp; hairline involved
■ **Atopic dermatitis**	Typical lesions elsewhere; pruritic; scalp lesions more diffuse
■ **Alopecia areata**	Circular or oval lesions without scale or inflammation
■ **Aplasia cutis congenita**	Patch of alopecia since birth; no scale or inflammation
■ **Trichotillomania**	Irregular patches with hair of different lengths, grows evenly when shaved

Table 48. Systemic treatment of tinea capitis

Agent	Dosage	Duration
■ **Griseofulvin**	10 mg/kg (up to 20–40 mg/kg) once daily after meal	8 weeks (often 16–24 weeks)
■ **Itraconazole**	5 mg/kg (liquid) <20 kg → 50 mg >20 kg → 100 mg once daily with main meal	4 weeks (–8 weeks)
■ **Terbinafine***	<20 kg → 62.5 mg 20–40 kg → 125 mg >40 kg → 250 mg once daily	4 weeks (–8 weeks)

* in case of *Microsporum canis* doubling of dosage recommended

ly dosage of 15–20 mg/kg is usually chosen. While a treatment period of at least 8 weeks is suggested, in clinical practice treatment for 4–6 months is often needed.

Two far more effective agents, itraconazole (an azole) and terbinafine (an allylamine), have shown documented superiority to griseofulvin especially regarding the length of treatment in several studies and are also safe in children. For this reason, we have not prescribed griseofulvin for a number of years for children. Both of the newer agents usually cure the patient with four to eight weeks of treatment (Table 48). One must carefully counsel the parents and document this, as these agents are not officially approved for children. Fluconazole is approved for systemic fungal infections (candidiasis, cryptococcosis) in children >1 year of age, but not for treatment of dermatophyte infections. There is very limited data on the efficacy of fluconazole in the treatment of tinea capitis.

Figure 56 shows our approach to the treatment of tinea capitis. Once the diagnosis is made, we treat for 4 weeks with itraconazole 5 mg/kg daily due to the superiority of this drug against *Microsporum*, the leading cause of tinea capitis in our clinic. In addition a topical antifungal agent with another mechanism of action is used simultaneously (e.g., topical allylamine or ciclopiroxolamine in the case of systemic azole, topical ciclopiroxolamine or azole in the case of systemic terbinafine).

Clinical examination is not adequate to determine if a cure has been achieved. One must employ KOH exam and fungal culture. The patient is re-examined two weeks after finishing the systemic treatment, and again after two more weeks. If on both occasions, the fungal culture is negative, we regard the child as cured. Sometimes the KOH is positive on the first re-check, but the culture is negative; this is not an indication for re-treatment. If the dermatophyte is identified again on culture, we retreat for just two weeks.

In our hands, a four week course of itraconazole cures 96% of the cases of tinea capitis not caused by *Microsporum canis*; for those caused by *Microsporum canis*, the cure rate is 88%. While terbinafine is also very effective in *Trichophyton* tinea capitis, cure rates are lower in *Microsporum* tinea capitis.

■ **Side Effects.** Both itraconazole and terbinafine are safe drugs and no laboratory studies are mandatory. Occasionally children complain of mild gastrointestinal distress or headache mostly resolving spontaneously after a short period of time. The main concern with itraconazole and terbinafine is hepatotoxicity; it is therefore not used in patients with impaired liver function or previous drug-induced hepatitis. When itraco-

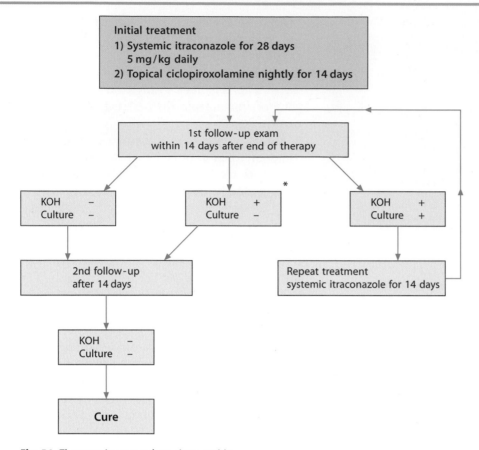

Fig. 56. Therapeutic approach to tinea capitis.

nazole is prescribed, one cannot simultaneously employ terfenadine, astemizole or erythromycin and other drugs metabolized by cytochrome P450-3A4, because of the risk of cardiac rhythm disturbances with ventricular extrasystoles. Terbinafine can alter serum levels of cimetidine, some antidepressants and warfarin. Exanthems are rare, but probably slightly more frequent and more severe with terbinafine.

■ **Supportive Measures.** In addition to employing a topical antifungal cream as discussed above, we ask the child to wash their hair every other day for the first two weeks with a shampoo containing an antifungal agent (e.g., selenium sulfide, ketoconazole, ciclopiroxolamine).

The infected child should not share combs, hair brushes, wash clothes, towels or headgear with anyone else. The child can continue to go to school once therapy has been instituted. If weeping lesions are present, it may be wiser to keep the child at home for a few days with aggressive treatment.

One should also search for the source of infection. Household pets, even asymptomatic ones, should be checked by a veterinarian; cats with *Microsporum canis* are often asymptomatic. For pets, there is a vaccine which can be used prophylactically and therapeutically against all important dermatophyte infections. Other family members, especially those sharing headgear, pillows, and the like, should also be screened closely.

■ **Treatment of Kerion.** In the case of a kerion, the antifungal treatment alone is usually not adequate. Anti-inflammatory measures are also required. We use a topical corticosteroid cream or solution b.i.d. for the first 3–5 days;

a kerion is one clinical setting where a combination corticosteroid/antibiotic or corticosteroid/antifungal product may be useful. In those children with fever and lymphadenopathy, we sometimes also give a burst of systemic corticosteroids (methylprednisolone 1.0 mg/kg daily for 3 days, followed by 0.5 mg/kg for the next 3 days) along with the oral antimycotic agent. In very inflammatory disease, there may be significant bacterial superinfection. Most cases only need topical treatment with antiseptics, but sometimes a course of oral antibiotics is indicated.

References

Degreef H.: The changing spectrum of tinea capitis. Current Opinion in Dermatology 3:44–48 (1996)

Friedlander S.F., Aly R., Krafchik B., Blumer J., Honig P., Steward D., Lucky A.W., Gupta A.K., Babel D.E., Abrams B., Gourmala N., Wraith L., Paul C. and the Tinea capitis Study Group: Terbinafine in the treatment of Trichophyton tinea capitis: a randomized, double-blind, parallel-group, duration-finding study. Pediatrics 109:602–607 (2002)

Ginter G.: Microsporum canis infections in children: results of a new oral antifungal therapy. Mycoses 39:265–269 (1996)

Gupta A.K., Ginter G: Itraconazole is effective in the treatment of tinea capitis caused by Microsporum canis. Pediatr Dermatol 18:519–522 (2001)

Herbert A.A.: Diagnosis and treatment of tinea capitis in children. Dermatologic Therapy 2:78–83 (1997)

Higgins E.M., Fuller L.C., Smith C.H.: Guidelines for the management of tinea capitis. British Journal of Dermatology 143:53–58 (2000)

Koumantaki E., Georgala S., Rallis E., Papadavid E.: Microsporum canis tinea capitis in an 8-month-old infant successfully treated with 2 weekly pulses of oral itraconazole. Pediatric Dermatology 18:60–62 (2001)

Lipozencic J., Skerlev M., Orofino-Costa R., Zaitz V.C., Horvath A., Chouela E., Romero G., Gourmala N., Paul C., and the Tinea capitis Study Group: A randomized, double-blind, parallel-group, duration-finding study of oral terbinafine and open-label, high-dose griseofulvin in children with tinea capitis due to Microsporum species. Br J Dermatol 146:816–823 (2002)

Mercurio M.G., Elewski B.: Tinea capitis treatment. Dermatologic Therapy 3:79–83 (1997)

Möhrenschlager M., Schnopp C., Fesq H., Strom K., Beham A., Mempel M., Thomsen S., Brockow K., Wessner D.B., Heidelberger A., Ruhdorfer S., Weigl L., Seidl H.P., Ring J., Abeck D.: Optimizing the therapeutic approach in tinea capitis of childhood. British Journal of Dermatology 143:1011–1015 (2000)

Richardson M.D., Warnock D.M.: Fungal infections. Diagnosis and management, 2nd. ed. Blackwell Science, Oxford (1997)

Suarez S., Friedlander S.F.: Antifungal therapy in children: an update. Pediatric Annals 27:177–184 (1998)

CHAPTER 22 Urticaria

K. BROCKOW

Epidemiology

Urticaria is one of the most common skin diseases in children. Girls are more often affected than boys. The exact incidence is not known, but it is estimated that 20% of children experience at least one episode of hives before reaching adulthood.

Pathogenesis

Hives are the result of capillary leakage with tissue swelling (edema) and erythema due to excessive release of proinflammatory mediators after non-specific (and often unknown) stimuli. Included in the list of possible trigger factors are infections (viral, bacterial, parasitic), medications, foods, food additives, physical factors, autoimmune diseases, and malignancies. In children, infections are the most common cause. In one analysis of 76 cases, infections were identified in 60%, drug reactions in 10% and food intolerance in 5%. In only 17% of cases was no likely cause found. In another study of 75 children with chronic urticaria, once again infections were the most common cause (36%), followed by food intolerance reactions (33%), inhalation allergies, and medications. Physical urticaria caused by mechanical factors (pressure, rubbing) or thermal (heat, cold) is less common in children than adults. In our personal experience, once infections have been excluded, about half the children with chronic urticaria have no discernible cause, even after extensive investigations.

Clinical Features

Urticaria is characterized by the presence of hives or wheals. While individual hives are short-lived (usually less than 24 hours), lesions continuously develop so that many lesions are often present simultaneously. Hives can vary greatly in their appearance and number. They can be small, isolated erythematous papules, or larger plaques covering large areas of the body (Fig. 57). They may intersect and coalesce causing annular, gyrate or map-like patterns (Fig. 58). If the edema is deeper, the skin changes may be minimal or non-existent, and instead only a swelling is seen, known as angioedema or urticaria profunda (Fig. 59). In about 50% of cases, angioedema is associated with urticaria and can be viewed as a deep variant; in the other cases hives are not seen. An example of the latter is hereditary angioedema caused by an inherited deficiency or functional defect in the C1-esterase inhibitor. Patients with severe urticaria and particularly with angioedema may have other signs and symptoms of anaphylaxis.

Urticaria is divided into acute (present <6 weeks) and chronic (present >6 weeks). Chronic urticaria can then be further classified as chronic recurrent with disease-free intervals of more than one day; and chronic-continuous, when the child is never free of hives for 24 hours. Acute urticaria is much more common and often resolves spontaneously. Chronic urticaria is uncommon in young children, but seen more often in older children and adolescents.

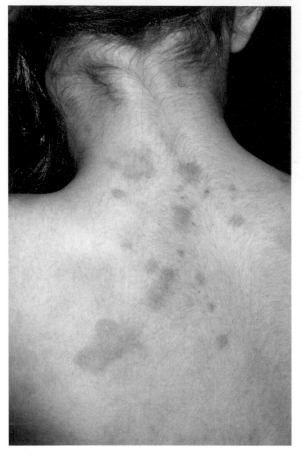

Fig. 57. Acute urticaria. Disseminated erythematous papules and plaques.

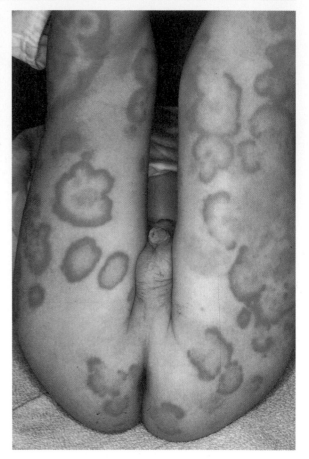

Fig. 58. Acute urticaria. Annular lesions following resolution of central component.

Symptoms

The classic symptom of urticaria is pruritus which can be intense. Since hives are more common in the evening and early morning hours, they may lead to sleep disturbances.

Diagnosis

The clinical diagnosis of urticaria is easy; hives are a snap diagnosis. Most often the parent or child even says "I have hives." The most important question is how long the individual lesions persist. The evaluation of a child with hives in order to determine the etiology is much more complex. The most important aspect is a detailed history, inquiring about ato-

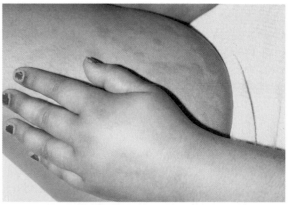

Fig. 59. Deep urticaria. Skin colored swelling of the back of the hand without obvious hives.

py, previous "allergic" reactions, medications, recent dietary history, and the circumstances associated with the development of the hives. In the case of acute urticaria, screening labo-

Table 49. Diagnostic approach to urticaria

1. Routine evaluation in chronic urticaria and in selected cases of acute urticaria

- History
- Physical examination
- Routine laboratory tests (CBC, sed rate, IgE level, stool for ova and parasites; C1 INH and C4 in selected cases)
- Physical testing (dermographism, pressure, warm, cold, exercise)
- Allergy testing (prick testing with standard allergens)
- Avoidance of suspicious medications

2. More intensive search in chronic urticaria

Diary with diet, activities, and record of urticaria

Search for focus of infection	Dental and ENT examinations; abdominal sonography; chest X-ray
Laboratory	Culture and serology (viruses, bacteria, fungi); ANA; cryoglobulins; cold agglutinins; serum protein electrophoresis; thyroid function tests; electrolytes, BUN, creatinine
Allergy testing	Extended prick testing; RAST; perhaps direct application of suspected foods and medications to skin

3. Provocation when suspicious of food allergy

- Elimination diet; followed by gradual reintroduction of foods
- Provocation tests with foods and food additives (in hospital, ideally double blind, placebo controlled)

Table 50. Differential diagnosis of urticaria

Diagnosis	Distinguishing Features
■ **Urticarial vasculitis**	Individual lesions persist more than 24 hours; often purpuric in center; patients usually have fever, arthralgias, other signs of systemic disease
■ **Erythema multiforme**	Target lesions, often acral, with urticarial border and livid or bullous center
■ **Erythema marginatum**	Transient faint annular to polycyclic erythematous lesions associated with rheumatic fever; non-pruritic
■ **Erythema annulare centrifugum**	Annular erythematous lesions with peripheral scale; persist for days to weeks; non-pruritic
■ **Urticaria pigmentosa**	Disseminated red-brown macules and papules; rubbing causes them to swell and become urticarial (Darier sign); caused by infiltrates of mast cells (Chap. 13)
■ **Hereditary angioedema**	Usually familial; only angioedema without urticaria; non-pruritic; often gastro-intestinal complaints

same applies to cholinergic urticaria. Physical testing can be done to confirm the diagnosis and obtain baseline values useful in monitoring treatment and the course of the disease.

A helpful step is to have the patient and parents keep a diary, including foods, medications, activities and the occurrence and severity of hives. This inexpensive measure often guides the physician into ordering the right tests to solve the mystery of the hives.

Differential Diagnosis

The differential diagnostic considerations for urticaria are shown in Table 50. Urticarial vasculitis is frequently discussed, but rarely seen in children. Classic patients have complement abnormalities, arthritis and renal disease as well as persistent hives. Dermatologists have come to biopsy any patient with individual hives lasting more than 24 hours; however, since this phenomenon is relatively common in ordinary hives, the yield of a biopsy is low.

ratory measures are not cost effective and should not be employed. If there are other signs and symptoms of an infection, the appropriate confirmatory tests (for example, hepatitis serology) should be obtained. If a reaction to a medication or foodstuff is suspected, then the product should be avoided and once the hives have cleared, the patient is best referred for allergy testing.

In the case of chronic urticaria, the workup is lengthier as shown in Table 49.

Physical urticaria can present as urticarial dermographism, pressure urticaria or cold urticaria. In these cases careful history-taking usually gives the clue to the diagnosis; the

Therapy

■ **Acute Urticaria and Angioedema.** Mild cases of urticaria require no treatment or perhaps a non-sedating H1 antihistamine such as cetirizine or loratadine. If an antihistamine is prescribed, the patient should take it regularly for 10–14 days, not just when hives appear. Once hives have been suppressed for this time period, the vast majority have already disappeared and the treatment is ended.

Topical antipruritic measures may also be helpful. We prefer polidocanol 5–10% in a zinc shake lotion. Topical corticosteroids are frequently prescribed but they are not especially effective antipruritic agents and are far more expensive.

If the hives are more severe, we switch to a sedating antihistamine, usually dimethindene maleate. In severe cases, we add methylprednisolone 1 mg/kg daily for a few days.

If the patient has signs and symptoms of asthma or anaphylaxis, more aggressive treatment is required. Both the dimethindene maleate and prednisolone (2–5 mg/kg) are administered intravenously, along with epinephrine (1:1000, diluted 1:10 in saline, then 0.1 mL/kg preferably i.v.; may be repeated after 20 minutes; maximum dosage 5 mL).

■ **Hereditary Angioedema.** Acute attacks are treated with C1-esterase inhibitor (1000–2000 IU), fresh plasma infusion (400–2000 mL), intravenous fluids and airway control. For prophylaxis before a surgical or dental procedure, either C1-esterase inhibitor or aminocaproic acid is employed, while for long-term prophylaxis, the synthetic androgens danazol and stanazol, as well as aminocaproic acid, are usually chosen. Because of possible long-term side effects, cooperation with a pediatric endocrinologist or gynecologist is necessary.

■ **Chronic Urticaria.** The ideal treatment for urticaria is identifying and eliminating the responsible triggering factor. Since this is

Table 51. Treatment of chronic urticaria

- Identification and elimination of trigger
- Non-sedating antihistamines
- Addition of sedating antihistamines, alone or in combination
- Combination of H1 and H2 antihistamines
- Addition of β-sympathomimetic agents
- Systemic corticosteroids (rarely needed)

accomplished in less than 50% of cases, the majority of patients require symptomatic therapy. One must remember that, perhaps because of the many different causes, the individual response to various therapeutic regimens is highly variable, so that an ideal approach is usually the result of many different attempts and adjustments (Table 51).

Oral antihistamines are the mainstay (see Appendix III). Continuous usage is better than trying to take the medication only when hives occur, as in general they are far more effective at preventing histamine-induced reactions than in treating them. Tachyphylaxis can develop, so it is often wise to have the patient switch products occasionally.

In school-age children, we use non-sedating antihistamines, such as cetirizine or loratadine, in order not to interfere with their school and homework. If these are unsatisfactory, sedating antihistamines such as dimethindene maleate and clemastine can be employed. They should also be used at bedtime. The range of both tolerated and effective levels is wide, so that one should start at a low dosage and gradually increase it.

The most common side effect of the older antihistamines is sedation, but in small children there may be a paradoxical CNS stimulation with agitation, insomnia, and tremor. This untoward reaction requires discontinuation of the medication. Other side effects such as gastrointestinal signs and symptoms (nausea, vomiting, diarrhea), headache and anticholinergic problems (dry mouth, cardiac arrhythmias) can be seen in children, usually when the dosage is too high or when the metabolism of the drug in the liver is reduced, either by liver disease or by use of other cytochrome P450-metabolized agents such as imidazole antifungals or macrolide antibiotics.

■ **Other Therapeutic Possibilities.** When single antihistamines are not effective, one can combine two different H1 blockers, increase the dose or add an H2 blocker, such as cimetidine. While some studies suggest that the combination is clearly more effective, others have failed to confirm this advantage. The main side effects of H2 antihistamines include interactions with cytochrome P450-metabolized drugs, as well as gynecomastia and azoospermia. The tricylic antidepressant doxepin possesses both H1 and H2 actions; it can be used in children older than 12 years of age in dosages of 25–50 mg daily. The side effects are multiple, including dry mouth, constipation, and fatigue. Ketotifen (maximum dose 1 mg b.i.d. in children 2–10 years and 2 mg b.i.d. in children >10 years) also has both H1 and H2 blocking actions.

Another possibility is β-sympathomimetic agents such as terbutaline (0.5–0.75 mg b.i.d. in infants <2 years, 0.75–1.5 mg b.i.d. in children 2–6 years and 1.5–3 mg b.i.d. in children 7–14 years) which can be used with H1 antihistamines or ketotifen. Subcutaneous terbutaline (0.05 mg b.i.d. in infants <2 years, 0.1 mg b.i.d. in children 2–6 years and 0.15 mg b.i.d. in children 7–14 years of age) is more effective than the oral form.

Cromolyn and other mast cell stabilizers are not effective in chronic urticaria. Oral corticosteroids should not be routinely used in treating urticaria. In totally unresponsive cases, one can treat with methylprednisolone 0.5 mg/kg daily for no more than 7 days, switching then to alternative day treatment and tapering the dose over a few weeks.

■ **Physical Urticaria.** Physical urticaria is treated by avoiding the physical triggers. Some patients demonstrate hardening when they are gradually exposed to increasing amounts of the physical trigger. Prophylactic antihistamines may be helpful. In the case of cold urticaria, cyprohepatidine may be more effective than other agents in a dosage of 2–4 mg t.i.d. One unpleasant side effect is an increase in appetite and weight gain. Hydroxyzine is perhaps superior to the other agents in treating cholinergic urticaria. In urticarial dermographism, either H1 blockers or the combination of H1 and H2 blockers usually reduce the extent of the reaction. Solar urticaria can be treated with both antihistamines and light-induced hardening with UVA, UVA1, UVB, or PUVA. Pressure urticaria is often not responsive to antihistamines and may occasionally require systemic corticosteroids.

References

Black A.K., Greaves M.W.: Antihistamines in urticaria and angioedema. Clin Allergy Immunol 17:249–286 (2002)

Charlesworth E.N.: Urticaria and angioedema: a clinical spectrum. Annals of Allergy, Asthma and Immunology 76:484–495 (1996)

Greaves M.: Chronic urticaria. Journal of Allergy and Clinical Immunology 105:664–672 (2000)

Farkas H., Harmat G., Fust G., Varga L., Visy B.: Clinical management of hereditary angio-oedema in children. Pediatr Allergy Immunol 13:153–161 (2002)

Halpern S.R.: Chronic hives in children: analysis of 75 cases. Annals of Allergy 23:589–599 (1965)

Juhlin L., Landor M.: Drug therapy for chronic urticaria. Clinical Reviews in Allergy 10:349–369 (1992)

La Rosa M., Leopardi S., Marchese G., Corrias A., Barberio G., Oggioan N., Grimaldi I.: Double-blind multicenter study on the efficacy and tolerability of cetirizine compared with oxatomide in chronic idiopathic urticaria in preschool children. Ann Allergy Asthma Immunol 87:48–53 (2001)

Schuller D.E.: Acute urticaria in children. Postgraduate Medicine 72:179–185 (1982)

CHAPTER 23

Varicella-Zoster Virus Infections

A. HEIDELBERGER, H. CREMER

The varicella-zoster virus (VZV) is a DNA virus belonging to the herpes group. The initial infection with VZV causes varicella, also known as chickenpox. Following the healing of the varicella, the VZV remains in the body; its reactivation leads to zoster. VZV is the most infectious of all herpes viruses; at 12 years of age, more than 90% of children show serologic evidence of infection with VZV. Varicella may appear in epidemics; zoster tends to be a sporadic occurrence.

Varicella

Epidemiology

Varicella is a worldwide infection which was almost "obligatory" prior to the introduction of immunizations. 90% of the infections occur before 15 years of age (in the USA and Japan before 10 years of age). The peak age is between 2 and 6 years. In about 30% of cases, the infection occurs before 5 months of age, as the level of maternal antibodies against varicella transferred to the child gradually wane during the first four months.

Pathogenesis

Varicella is spread via airborne droplets via the respiratory tract. One needs almost direct contact with an infected child during the days when the virus is present in the nasal and oral secretions. The incubation period is up to four weeks, but averages two weeks. The child becomes infective 1–2 days before the appearance of the exanthem and remains infective until about the 6th day of the skin rash. Some colleagues consider varicella infective until all crusts have fallen off. Our rule is – infective until one day after last fresh blister appears. Until this point, children should be kept at home. They should in no case be allowed contact with immunosuppressed individuals (HIV/AIDS, cancer chemotherapy, hematological malignancies) or seronegative pregnant woman. On rare occasions, the droplets appear to spread over greater distances (gusts of wind, open windows), as a direct contact cannot be traced.

Clinical Features

Varicella is characterized by the appearance of crops of lesions, leading to a pattern where lesions in various stages of development are found close to one another (Fig. 60). This variability is known as a "star chart" in German, reflecting the varying nature of the skies as depicted in astronomy charts. It can be of critical importance, as in smallpox, all lesions tend to be in the same stage of development.

The initial lesions are erythematous macules which rapidly become papular and then over a matter of hours vesicular, producing small clear vesicles on a red base (Fig. 61). Later pustules and crusts form. The trunk is the main and usually first site of involvement. The face, scalp and limbs (centripetal spread) follow. The hands and feet are usually spared. Mucosa (mouth,

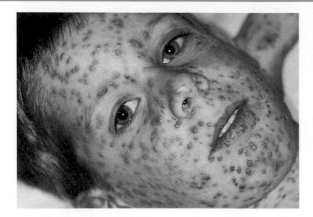

Fig. 60. Varicella. Many lesions in various stages including papules, papulo-vesicles and blisters.

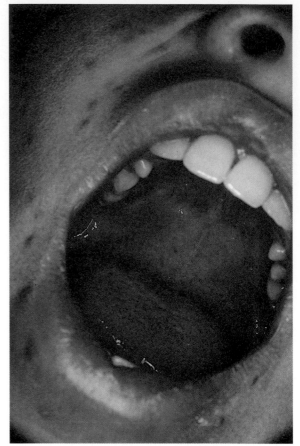

Fig. 62. Varicella. Punctate erythematous lesions on palate.

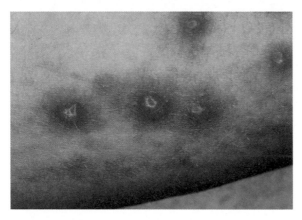

Fig. 61. Varicella. Vesicles on erythematous base.

eyes, genitalia) is frequently affected; the most typical lesions are erythematous macules and blisters on the hard palate (Fig. 62).

A peculiar feature of varicella is that it may be limited to areas of sun exposure, as well as other areas which are selectively irritated such as the diaper area or even at a site of immunization.

The ordinary lesions of varicella may scar but tend not to do so. The major complication is secondary infections with both staphylococci and streptococci, which then lead almost regularly to scarring, producing small round depressed scars. Other complications are more common in older patients than children and include pneumonia, hepatitis, encephalitis, and purpura fulminans.

A high risk scenario is the development of varicella in newborns, after the mother has been infected during the small time window of seven days before delivery to two days after delivery. In addition, newborns without adequate maternal protection, as well as immunosuppressed children, are at danger of experiencing severe cutaneous disease and internal complications.

Symptoms

The main symptom is pruritus. The scratching often contributes to the development of secondarily infected lesions. In the first three days of the infection, most children are febrile. Fever, malaise, nausea and headache are the typ-

Table 52. Differential diagnosis of varicella

Diagnosis	Distinguishing Features
■ Coxsackie virus infections	Usually maculo-papular; rarely vesicular; not pleomorphic
■ Eczema herpeticatum	Lesions all in the same stage; usually most prominent where pre-existing skin disease was worse (face, flexures for atopic dermatitis)
■ Smallpox	Lesions all in same stage; centrifugal spread with palms and soles involved; patient sick!

ical prodromal symptoms which may precede the exanthem; they are often more pronounced in older children and adults.

Diagnosis

The diagnosis can usually be made clinically, if it has not already been offered by the mother. One should always check the mouth and scalp when thinking of varicella. Occasionally identification of varicella zoster virus from fresh vesicles by direct immunofluorescence or PCR can be helpful to confirm the diagnosis.

Differential Diagnosis

The major differential diagnostic considerations are shown in Table 52.

Therapy

Symptomatic therapy is all that is needed for most children. Standard measures include antipyretics, adequate fluids and bland topical drying measures (usually zinc oxide shake lotion, perhaps with 1% chlorhexidine). Powders should not be used, as they are not designed for open, weeping lesions. In Germany, astringent baths with tannic acid derivatives are a popular adjunct.

The use of antiviral agents, primarily acyclovir, in varicella is modestly controversial. The major benefit in otherwise healthy children appears to be a slight shortening of the period of infectivity, which means a child can return to school sooner and, thus, a parent to work. Whether this societal benefit justifies treatment is a difficult decision. There is agreement that adolescents and adults should be treated, because there are more complications in this age group.

Depending on the severity of the disease, other measures may be needed (Table 53).

■ **High-risk Children.** Systemic antiviral agents should be considered in all immunosuppressed children, in hematological disease, and in children with chronic pulmonary disease, especially when on systemic corticosteroids.

In addition, some public health officials recommend active immunization in these children under certain circumstances (e.g., children with hematological disease in stable remission for at least 12 months, in children scheduled for renal transplantation).

VZ immune globulin is recommended as prophylaxis in high-risk patients (immunodeficient children, newborns, if the mother was infected between seven days before and two days after giving birth) when exposed to varicella (exposition defined as at least one hour contact in a room with face-to-face-contact or varicella infection of household member). VZ immune globulin has to be given within 96 hours after exposure.

Active immunization against varicella is not yet part of the official vaccination program for healthy children in most countries. There is preliminary data that active vaccination is also protective post-exposure when given within 36 hours.

One should contact local public health sources for the most recent, regionally relevant guidelines.

■ **Supportive Measures.** The patient should wear light clothing which breathes and does not rub. Excessive clothing produces warmth

Table 53. Treatment of varicella

1. Basic principles	– antipyretics (usually acetaminophen; never aspirin)
	– adequate fluids
	– antipruritic measures
2. Topical therapy of uncomplicated disease	
■ zinc oxide shake lotion	– with 5% polidocanol → antipruritic
	– with 1% chlorhexidine → antimicrobial
■ other non-toxic astringent lotions, such as calamine lotion (not Caldryl® which contains a topical antihistamine with high sensitizing potential) or tannic acid shake lotions	
■ cooling astringent baths; in Europe, tannic acid bath additives	
3. Secondary infections	
■ topical	– use of 1% chlorhexidine in shake lotion
	– aqueous gentian violet (0.25% skin, 0.1% mucosa)
	– fusidic acid cream
■ systemic	– penicillinase-resistant penicillin
	– first generation oral cephalosporin
4. Intense pruritus	
■ topical	– use of 5% polidocanol in shake lotion
	– may increase to 10% in children >6 years of age
■ systemic	sedating antihistamines (see Appendix III)

which worsens the pruritus. The fingernails should be cut short to reduce the likelihood of excoriations and secondary infections. The skin can be washed with lukewarm water without soap.

■ Zoster

Epidemiology

Zoster is a rare disease in children. In those under nine years of age, the incidence is 0.74/1000 yearly.

Pathogenesis

Zoster can only occur in children who have already had varicella. In most instances, the virus has remained latent in the child's neural tissue and is reactivated, rather than being the result of a second infection. It is unclear how much protection against zoster is provided by immunization. One speculation is that as more and more people are immunized, each of us is less likely to be exposed to VZV and receive less of a booster effect, thus, perhaps increasing the incidence of zoster.

Since some cases of varicella are not clinically recognized, the history is not always reliable. The most usual scenario is that a very young child still with maternal protection against VZV is exposed to the virus via a sibling and has a subclinical course. At the same time, the child fails to develop a strong immune response and is thus apparently more likely to develop zoster. Also at increased risk are immunosuppressed children, such as those with primary immunodeficiencies, HIV/AIDS or undergoing cancer chemotherapy.

Clinical Features

The classical pattern of zoster is the same clear vesicles on an erythematous back-

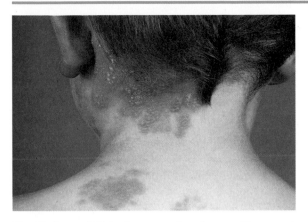

Fig. 63. Zoster. Unilateral segmental erythema with grouped, mainly clear vesicles.

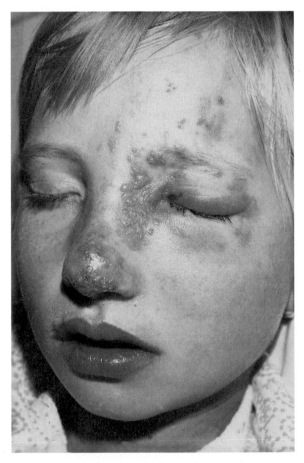

Fig. 64. Zoster. Involvement of first branch of trigeminal nerve with ocular and nasal involvement. Erythema, blisters and crusts.

ground as seen in varicella – but arranged in a dermatomal pattern involving just one segment of the body and almost always sparing the midline (Fig. 63). Facial involvement is not uncommon, often involving the trigeminal nerve (Fig. 64). If the nose is affected, the likelihood of ocular involvement is considerable, often leading to a keratitis. When the acoustic nerve is affected, there may be hearing disturbances, while facial nerve involvement can lead to paralysis. Generalized zoster is uncommon in children, but is a suggestion of inadequate immunity.

Symptoms

The typical complaint is localized pain or burning, often preceding any clinical signs by several days. Usually in children the skins lesions themselves are relatively asymptomatic and post-herpetic neuralgia is rare.

Diagnosis

The diagnosis can almost always be made clinically.

Differential Diagnosis

On occasion it can be difficult to separate zoster from herpes simplex. In such instances, immunofluorescent staining of the dried blister fluid can be used to identify either HSV or VZV. PCR can also be used to differentiate the two. Viral serologic studies can also be performed. Other differential diagnostic considerations are shown in Table 54.

Therapy

An uncomplicated zoster does not require the administration of acyclovir, especially in children. Our recommendations for the use of acyclovir in pediatric zoster are shown in Table 55. When ocular involvement is identi-

Varicella-Zoster
Virus Infections

Table 54. Differential diagnosis of zoster

Diagnosis	Distinguishing Features
■ **Herpes simplex**	Usually not dermatomal; recurs in same location
■ **Contact dermatitis (such as poison ivy)**	More pruritic; not dermatomal; history usually distinctive
■ **Erysipelas**	Localized erythema; not dermatomal; fever, chills, other systemic signs and symptoms
■ **Bullous arthropod bite reaction**	Intensely pruritic; not dermatomal; diascopy reveals punctate sites of bite or sting

Table 55. Indications for acyclovir in children

	Route of administration of acyclovir	
	Intact immunity	Reduced immunity
Location of zoster		
■ trunk, extremities	–	intravenous
■ ocular	oral	intravenous
■ otic	oral	intravenous

fied, usually in cooperation with an ophthalmologist, we also use acyclovir ophthalmic ointment and an wide spectrum antibiotic in an ophthalmic vehicle. Immunosuppressed patients should always be treated with systemic antiviral agents; we prefer the parenteral route.

Topical treatment is the same as for varicella; we use a zinc oxide shake lotion with 1% chlorhexidine added. Aqueous solutions of gentian violet are also helpful; 0.25% for the skin and 0.1% for the mucosa.

References

Arvin A.M.: Progress in the treatment and prevention of varicella. Current Opinion in Infectious Diseases 6:553–557 (1993)

Gold L., Barbour St., Guerrero-Tiro L., Koopot R., Lewis K., Rudinsky M., Williams R.: *Staphylococcus aureus* endocarditis associated with varicella infection in children. Pediatric Infectious Diseases Journal 15:377–379 (1996)

Hofmann F., Sydow B., Michaelis M.: Zur epidemiologischen Bedeutung von Varicellen. Gesundheitswesen 56:599–601 (1994)

Hurwitz S.: The exanthematous diseases of childhood, pp. 347–350. Clinical Pediatric Dermatology. W.B. Saunders, Philadelphia (1993)

Kakouru T., Theodoridou M., Mostrou G., Syriopoulou V., Papadogeorgaki H., Constantopoulos A.: Herpes zoster in children. Journal of the American Academy of Dermatology 39:207–210 (1998)

Klassen T.P., Belseck E.M., Wiebe N., Hartling L.: Acyclovir for treating varicella in otherwise healthy children and adolescents: a systematic review of randomized controlled trials. BMC Pediatr 2:9–17 (2002)

Magliocco A.M., Demetrich D.J., Sarnat H.B., Hwang W.S.: Varicella embryopathy. Archives of Pathology and Laboratory Medicine 116:181–186 (1992)

Shinefield H.R., Black S.B., Staehle B., Matthews H., Adelman T., Ensor K., Li S., Chan I., Heyse J., Waters M., Chan C.Y., Vessey S.J., Kaplan K.M., Kuter B.J., Kaiser Permanente Medical Team for Varivax: Pediatr Infect Dis J 21:555–561 (2002)

Smith C., Glaser A.: Herpes zoster in childhood: case report and review of the literature. Pediatric Dermatology 13:226–229 (1996)

Thomas S.L., Wheeler J.G., Hall A.J.: Contacts with varicella or with children and protection against herpes zoster in adults: a case-control study. Lancet 360:678–682 (2002)

Vugia D., Peterson C., Meyers H.B., Kim K.S., Arrieta A., Schlievert P., Kaplan E., Werner S.B., Mascola L.: Invasive group A streptococcal infections in children with varicella in Southern California. Pediatric Infectious Diseases Journal 15:146–150 (1996)

Watson B., Seward J., Yang A., Witte P., Lutz J., Chan C., Orlin S., Levenson R.: Postexposure effectiveness of varicella vaccine. Pediatrics 105:84–88 (2000)

CHAPTER 24 Vascular Anomalies

H. CREMER, S. THOMSEN

Introduction

Vascular anomalies include both vascular tumors and vascular malformations. In the past, these two different disease processes were often not firmly separated, but the recommendations of the International Society for the Study of Vascular Anomalies in 1996 make it clear that such a division is desirable for proper diagnostic and therapeutic measures.

Hemangiomas

The vast majority of vascular tumors in childhood are classical hemangiomas, which account for over 90% of all lesions. They are usually divided into superficial, deep and mixed forms. In addition, there are many rare variants which differ either in clinical or histological features and also have a different course or prognosis. In order to simplify this potentially complicated field, we will rely primarily on the clinical features for classification as shown in Table 56. We will concentrate on localized classical hemangiomas with reference to our own series of over 1000 cases.

Epidemiology

The incidence of hemangiomas has been estimated at 2–10%. In premature infants with a birth weight less than 1000 g, the incidence increases to as much as 30%. There is a female:male predominance of 3:1.

Pathogenesis

Hemangiomas are benign tumors of proliferating capillary endothelial cells. The cause of hemangiomas is unclear. A variety of angiogenesis factors are presumed to play a role, both *in utero* and after birth.

Clinical Features

About 85% of classical hemangiomas are superficial (usually bright red); 2%, deep (blue) and 13%, mixed. About 95% are solitary raised sharply circumscribed lesions (Fig. 65). Other much less common clinical variants include white hemangiomas (early precursor lesions) (Fig. 66), diffuse or large irregularly bordered hemangiomas (Fig. 67), agminate (grouped) hemangiomas (Fig. 68), and telangiectatic hemangiomas (Fig. 69). Table 56 shows a more detailed classification of hemangiomas.

Although hemangiomas are often not present at birth, at least 90% are visible by two months of age, often as bright red macules. It is impossible to predict the clinical course when initially assessing a hemangioma. Growth occurs readily over a matter of weeks or months reaching a plateau stage, typically between 6 and 9 months. At this point, about 70% of the tumors begin to regress; the first sign of regression being the net-like gray discoloration on the surface followed by flattening of the lesion. The superficial component usually resolves more rapidly than the deep. Sometimes areas of re-

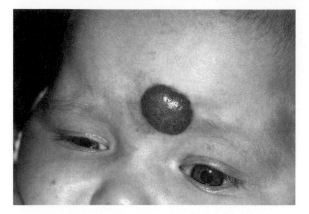

Fig. 65. Solitary hemangioma with well-defined border.

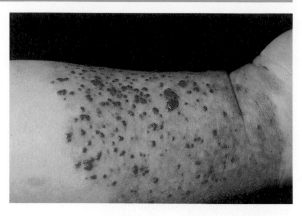

Fig. 68. Agminate hemangiomas.

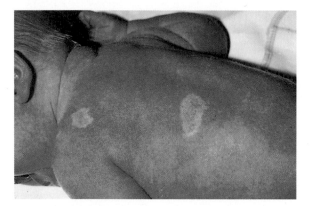

Fig. 66. White hemangioma.

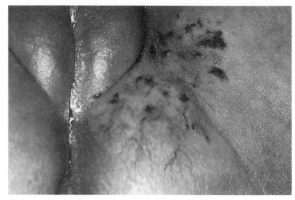

Fig. 69. Telangiectatic hemangioma.

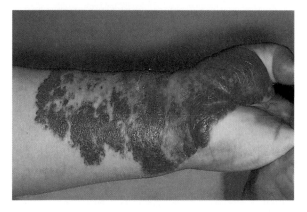

Fig. 67. Diffuse irregular hemangioma.

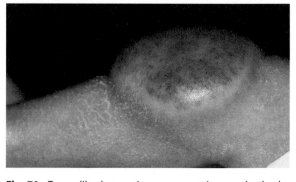

Fig. 70. Tumor-like hemangioma, present in completely developed form at birth.

gression are seen next to areas which are still growing, the mechanism of this phenomenon is not clear. Hemangiomas leave behind a variety of residual changes. These include telangiectases, fibrosis, hypopigmentation, and occasionally scarring from ulceration or as a result of more aggressive treatment. Some hemangiomas are fully present at birth but do not regress (Fig. 70); they are known as NICH (non-involuting congenital hemangiomas).

Important complications of hemangiomas occurring mainly in the rapid growth phase include impairment of function due to ob-

Table 56. Classification of hemangiomas

1. Classic localized hemangioma
  1.1 Superficial hemangioma (85% of total)
    1.1.1 Solitary well-circumscribed nodular hemangioma (95% of superficial lesions fall into this category)
    1.1.2 Hemangioma precursor (white hemangioma)
    1.1.3 Irregular diffuse plaque-like hemangioma
    1.1.4 Agminate hemangioma
    1.1.5 Telangiectatic hemangioma
  1.2 Deep hemangioma (2%)
  1.3 Combined hemangioma (13%)

2. Neonatal hemangiomatosis
  2.1 Benign neonatal hemangiomatosis
  2.2 Disseminated hemangiomatosis

3. Special types of hemangiomas
  3.1 Large hemangiomas in cranio-facial region (with or without visceral involvement)
  3.2 Hemangiomas in the neck/chin/lip region (with or without impaired breathing from associated upper airway lesions)
  3.3 Tumor-like hemangiomas of newborns which are fully developed at birth (Fig. 70)
    (a) fast involuting b) slow involuting c) non involuting ("NICH")

4. Hemangiomas combined with other malformations
  4.1 Lumbosacral hemangioma with tethered cord, urogenital malformations, lipomas of spinal canal and sacral irregularities
  4.2 Large facial hemangioma with posterior fossa malformation
  4.3 Other combinations

struction (eyes, nose), ulceration (anogenital area), infection (diaper area), high output cardiac failure (giant hemangiomas), and consumption coagulopathy through platelet trapping (Kasabach-Merritt syndrome) most often associated with kaposiform hemangioendothelioma. Hemangiomas in rapid growth phase should be monitored very regularly, preferably with exact measurements and/or photographs to initiate treatment before complications occur.

Diagnosis

Typical hemangiomas can be diagnosed at a glance, if the parents (or grandparents) have not already made the diagnosis. Large or deep hemangiomas, as well as those in problem areas should be imaged using ultrasonography, Doppler ultrasonography or magnetic resonance imaging. If embolization with a subsequent operation is planned, then angiography must also be performed.

Differential Diagnosis

The major differential diagnostic considerations for distinguishing between vascular tumors and malformations are shown in Table 57.

Therapy

The approach to treating hemangiomas in infants has changed dramatically in recent years. Both the introduction of a variety of effective measures and an increased appreciation for the psychosocial impact of hemangiomas have contributed to this trend. Today early treatment is recommended for:

■ Hemangiomas in cosmetically critical areas (face)
■ Hemangiomas in problem areas, such as periocular (visual problems, including blindness), lips (feeding difficulties and tendency not to regress), nose (permanent distortion), and anogenital region (frequent ulcerations) (Fig. 71)
■ Rapidly growing tumors at any site

In general, the earlier a hemangioma is treated, the better the results. Most treatments can be performed on an ambulatory basis. The goal of therapy is not the destruction of the hemangioma, but instead arresting the growth phase and inaugurating the regression phase. The choice of the optimal approach depends on the size, depth, and growth rate of the lesion as well as the experience of the treating physician.

■ **Contact Cryotherapy.** This method is the one with which we have the most experience. It is ideally suited to treating those 95% of he-

Vascular Anomalies

Table 57. Differential diagnosis of hemangiomas and vascular malformations

Hemangioma	Vascular malformation
■ Ratio w:m 3:1	■ Ratio w:m 1:1
■ Appear days to weeks after birth	■ Present at birth, but may become more obvious later
■ Initial rapid growth	■ Growth proportional to that of body
■ Later regression	■ No regression
■ Proliferating endothelium with increased numbers of mast cells	■ Normal to dilated vessels, sometimes with shunts
■ Angiography shows feeding vessels and intense parenchymal staining	■ Angiography shows differences between high and low flow areas, no parenchymal staining

mangiomas which are single well-defined raised lesions. One can either employ metal rods cooled with $-196\,^{\circ}C$ with liquid N_2 which are applied with measured pressure to the hemangioma for 5–10 seconds, or electrical devices with Peltier elements which reach $-32\,^{\circ}C$ and thus must be applied for 15–20 seconds. The endothelial cells surrounding the blood are destroyed during freezing, while the less vascular epidermis and connective tissue are relatively spared. Thus, in most cases, scarring can be avoided. Freezing for too long or using a cryospray device are the two most likely causes of scarring. When freezing moist areas, the metal rod must be continuously turned to avoid it becoming stuck to the skin. No anesthesia is needed for smaller lesions; for larger hemangiomas, pre-operative use of EMLA cream under occlusion for 45–60 minutes provides good pain relief. A single treatment usually suffices; if not, the procedure is repeated at four week intervals.

■ **Flashlamp Pumped Dye Laser (FPDL).** This laser provides energy at a wave length (585 nm) which is almost completely absorbed by hemoglobin and, thus, produces selective photothermolysis of cutaneous vessels. The depth of penetration is only 2 mm. Although the FPDL is the treatment of choice for superficial vascular malformations, it is also very useful for superficial hemangiomas. It is a very safe method and used by some as a first choice for superficial hemangiomas in the face and diaper region. The only side effect is occasional post-inflammatory hypo- or hyperpigmentation.

■ **Neodymium-YAG Laser.** The Nd-YAG laser works on a completely different principle as the FPDL. Its 1064 nm waves can penetrate to a depth of 7 mm, allowing it to work on deeper hemangiomas not reached by contact cryotherapy or the FPDL. The skin is usually cooled with an ice cube through which the laser beam is directed. This protects the superficial layers. More elegant cooling devices are also available. The treatment is painful so that general anesthesia is usually required. The laser field is changing so rapidly that the reader is best advised to check the latest literature for additional information.

■ **Plastic Surgery.** Primary surgical excision of a hemangioma is rarely appropriate. The major indication is large tumors in the periocular region, especially the lids, which are blocking vision. On the other hand, plastic surgery is used to repair residual defects.

■ **Corticosteroids and Interferon-α 2 a.** Sometimes more aggressive systemic therapy is required in life-threatening situations. Examples include the Kasabach-Merritt syndrome with a consumptive coagulopathy, disseminated hemangiomas with internal complications, and hemangiomas which are threatening vision, airway patency or other vital functions but are not amenable to surgery or laser treatment. In such instances, systemic corticosteroids are recommended in dosages of methylprednisolone ranging from 2–3 up to 5 mg/kg daily over a period of 6–12 weeks. Responsive hemangiomas will show signs of regression after 1–2 weeks. If the patient fails to respond, another possibility is interferon-α 2 a (3 million IU/m^2 weekly), sometimes combined with corticosteroids. Both of these approaches have considerable side effects and should only be administered in centers with experience in their use.

Vascular Malformations

Vascular malformations are lesions caused by vascular or lymphatic dysmorphogenesis or aberrant embryological formation of capillary vessels. They are classified according to the vessel type. Capillary malformations are the most common, occurring in 0.3% of children. Venous malformations are less frequent, followed by lymphatic malformations of different vessel size (simple, cavernous). They are often unilateral, most common in the head and neck region and may be associated with similar malformations in other organs. They are usually present at birth and do not undergo a rapid growth phase but instead grow proportionally with the rest of the body.

Clinical Features

The most common anomaly is the stork bite (also known as nevus flammeus neonatorum or salmon patch). The pink-red lesions on the nape tend to be permanent while those on the glabella tend to fade away. They most likely represent functionally dilated vessels, rather than malformations and are not associated with underlying disorders.

The other lesions are true malformations and permanent; their most common name is port wine stain or nevus flammeus. A port wine stain is initially bright red but acquires a livid color worthy of its name; in adults nodules of localized vascular proliferation may arise within the flat patch.

The port wine stains can be associated with malformations of deeper vessels including venous, arteriovenous and even lympha-

tic lesions with dilatation and shunting. The red-blue arteriovenous malformations are not always identified at birth but increase in size as the child grows and often develop shunts. The various associations have been given a variety of names:

- In Sturge-Weber syndrome, a nevus flammeus involves the part of the face innervated by the trigeminal nerve. There may be leptomeningeal involvement (seizures, mental retardation) or ocular changes including glaucoma. When the first branch of the trigeminal nerve (V-1) is involved the risk of systemic involvement or glaucoma is about 75%. If V-2 or V-3 is affected, the chances are much lower.
- Klippel-Trénaunay syndrome combines a port wine stain of an extremity, more often a leg, with underlying deep vascular malformations often resulting in shunting, overgrowth of the limb (on rare occasion, growth retardation) and even high output cardiac failure.
- von Hippel-Lindau syndrome combines usually insignificant cutaneous lesions with retinal and cerebellar vascular changes as well as renal cysts and tumors, along with a variety of other malformations.

Diagnosis

The diagnosis of the cutaneous lesion is straight forward. Imaging studies are needed to accurately assess possible deep or systemic involvement. This should be undertaken before 3 years of age.

Differential Diagnosis

While the clinical diagnosis of a vascular malformation is usually straight-forward, Table 58 lists some of the lesions which can confused with hemangiomas and vascular malformations.

Vascular Anomalies

Table 58. Other lesions that can be confused with hemangiomas and vascular malformations

Diagnosis	Comments
■ Pyogenic granuloma (eruptive angioma)	Not present at birth; sudden development of eroded or deep red nodules; usually face or hands; surface often eroded or crusted and friable; can regress spontaneously
■ Tufted angioma	Flat bruise-like lesion, usually on head or upper trunk; slowly spreading; do not regress; while present in children, rarely seen at birth; rarely associated with Kasabach-Merritt syndrome
■ Kaposiform hemangioendothelioma	Nodular or infiltrative vascular tumors often present at birth or in first 2 years; do not regress; can be locally aggressive; the tumor most often associated with Kasabach-Merritt syndrome

Table 59. Treatment of hemangiomas and vascular malformations

Method	Indication	Comments
■ Contact cryotherapy	Superficial solitary hemangiomas, ulcerated hemangiomas	Epidermis spared; little risk of necrosis
■ Flashlamp pumped dye laser	Superficial hemangiomas, may induce regression in deeper hemangiomas; port wine stains	Little thermal damage because of short pulse duration
■ Nd:YAG laser (superficial)	Flat to nodular hemangiomas; may induce regression in deeper hemangiomas	Increased risk of scarring; ice cooling needed for deeper lesions
■ Nd:YAG laser (interstitial)	Large, deep hemangiomas	Can reduce risk of hemorrhage, also as pre-operative measure
■ Embolization	Large deep hemangiomas or vascular malformations	Can reduce risk of hemorrhage, also as pre-operative measure
■ Excision	Impairment of vital structures; lesions which are located at a site favorable for surgery	Rapid treatment but always scarring
■ Systemic corticosteroids	Life-threatening hemangiomas, including those with complications (blindness, Kasabach-Merritt syndrome)	Multiple steroid side effects and possible growth retardation
■ Interferon-α 2 a	Life-threatening hemangiomas, including those with complications (blindness, Kasabach-Merritt syndrome); failure to respond to corticosteroids	Many side effects; differing opinions about effectiveness

Therapy

Port wine stains are cosmetically disturbing. Since they are easiest to treat when the vessels are smaller, the standard approach is photothermolysis with the FPDL during the first year of life. Facial lesions respond much better to laser therapy than do port wine stains of the trunk or extremities. The goal is not total elimination of the blemish, but an marked lightening.

Deeper lesions may be amenable to vascular surgical intervention in specialized centers. This intervention is usually delayed until three years of age.

Stork bites require no treatment.

References

Achauer B.M., Chang C.J., Vander-Kam V.M. Management of hemangioma of infancy: review of 245 patients. Plastic Reconstructive Surgery 99: 1301–1308 (1997)

Barlow R.J., Walker N.P.J., Markey A.C.: Treatment of proliferative hemangiomas with the 585 nm pulsed dye laser. British Journal of Dermatology 134:700–704 (1996)

Cooper J.G., Edward S.L., Holmes J.D.: Kaposiform haemangioendothelioma: case report and review of the literature. Br J Plast Surg 55:163–165 (2002)

Cremer H., Djawari D.: Hämangiomtherapie. Der Kinderarzt 27:491–499 (1996)

Cremer H.: Vascular Tumors (Hemangiomas) in Childhood: in Chang J.B. (ed.), Textbook of Angiology. Springer New York (2000)

Ezekowitz R.A.B., Mulliken J.B., Folkmann J.: Interferon α 2a for life threatening hemangiomas of infancy. New England Journal of Medicine 326:1456–1463 (1992)

Gangopadhyay A.N., Sinha C.K., Gopal S.C., Gupta D.K., Sahoo S.P., Ahmad M.: Role of steroids in childhood hemangioma: a 10 year review. International Surgery 82:49–51 (1997)

Hohenleutner U., Bäumler W., Karrer S., Michel S., Landthaler M.: Die Behandlung kindlicher Hämangiome mit dem blitzlampengepumpten gepulsten Farbstofflaser. Hautarzt 47:183–189 (1996)

Kautz G., Cremer H. (Hrsg.) Hämangiome. Diagnostik und Therapie in Bild und Text. Springer, Berlin, Heidelberg, New York (1999)

Qu Z., Liebler J.M., Powers M.R., Galey T., Ahmadi P., Huang X.N., Ansel J.C., Butterfield J.H., Planck S.R., Rosenbaum J.T.: Mast cells are a major source of basic fibroblast growth factor in chronic inflammation and cutaneous hemangioma. Am J Pathol 147:564–573 (1995)

CHAPTER 25 Viral Exanthems

L. B. WEIGL

Gianotti-Crosti Syndrome

Epidemiology

Gianotti-Crosti syndrome is seen primarily in children between 1 and 6 years of age, with a maximum distribution of 3 months to 15 years. Patients tend to appear in clusters.

Pathogenesis

This syndrome is a post-viral reaction pattern, explaining the clustering as a reflection of viral patterns in the community. In the past, one distinguished between the true Gianotti-Crosti syndrome or papular acrodermatitis of childhood as a reflection of an underlying hepatitis B infection and papulovesicular acrolocated syndrome when other viral infections or no associated infection were found. Today, it is widely recognized, even in Gianotti and Crosti's famous clinic in Milan, that there is no difference.

The underlying virus simply reflect the nature of the community. In countries where hepatitis B infections are common in children, such as Korea, almost all cases are still caused by this virus. In Western Europe and America, the most common causes are probably Epstein-Barr virus and cytomegalovirus.

Clinical Features

The young patients are usually surprisingly well and have a monomorphic pattern of multiple red or red-brown papules and papulovesicles on the cheeks (Fig. 71), extensor aspects of the acral parts of the limbs (Fig. 72) and buttocks. Occasionally the lesions are hemorrhagic, and sometimes the palms and soles are involved. Only in exceptional cases is the trunk affected. The exanthem usually lasts 2 to 4 weeks, but may occasionally persist for 8 weeks.

Sometimes lymphadenopathy, hepatomegaly, or splenomegaly is seen, depending on the underlying virus. If hepatitis B virus is the cause, the patient is almost always anicteric, has a mild course, and rarely develops a chronic infection. The liver enzymes are slightly elevated and the hepatitis B-associated antigens can be identified either at the time of the rash or shortly thereafter.

Symptoms

The skin lesions are usually asymptomatic, but may occasionally be pruritic. Underlying symptoms reflecting the triggering viral infection are uncommon and can obviously be quite variable, but may include respiratory or gastrointestinal problems.

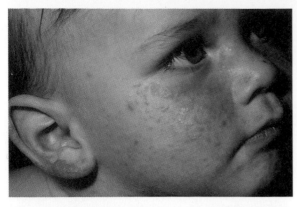

Fig. 71. Gianotti-Crosti syndrome. Many erythematous papules on cheek, chin and ear.

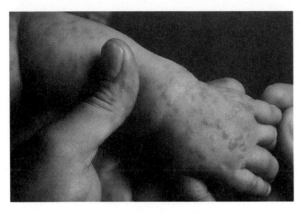

Fig. 72. Gianotti-Crosti syndrome. Multiple papules on extensor surface of forearm and back of hand.

Diagnosis

The diagnosis is usually clinically obvious. Serologic evaluation for hepatitis B virus should be performed, in order to be able to observe appropriate precautions and follow the patient for the unlikely development of a carrier status. Other viral tests may be needed, depending on the clinical picture.

Differential Diagnosis

The differential diagnostic considerations are listed in Table 60.

Table 60. Differential diagnosis of Gianotti-Crosti syndrome

Diagnosis	Distinguishing Features
■ **Lichen planus**	More intense pruritus; volar aspects of forearms most likely site; face rarely involved; Wickham striae (lacy white pattern) may been found on surface of large papules and on oral mucosa
■ **Lichenoid drug reaction**	History of exposure to medication; more pruritus, more diffuse disease
■ **Papular urticaria (strophulus)**	Marked pruritus; papules more urticarial; other family members involved; rapid improvement
■ **Erythema multiforme**	History of exposure to medications or herpes simplex virus; target-shaped lesions
■ **Urticaria**	Wheals, severe pruritus, rapidly changing clinical picture

Therapy

Usually no therapy is needed. If pruritus is a problem, topical corticosteroids may be useful. In more severe cases, systemic antihistamines or rarely systemic corticosteroids (short course of methylprednisolone 1 mg/kg daily tapered rapidly over 1 week) may be needed.

References

Boeck K., Mempel M., Schmidt T., Abeck D.: Gianotti-Crosti-syndrome: clinical, serologic and therapeutic data from nine children. Cutis 62:271–274 (1998)

Fölster-Holst R., Christophers E.: Exantheme im Kindesalter Teil 1: Exantheme durch Viren. Hautarzt 50:515–531 (1999)

Nelson J. S., Stone M. S.: Update on selected viral exanthems. Current Opinion in Pediatrics 12:359–364 (2000)

Mancini A. J.: Exanthems in childhood: An update. Pediatric Annals 27:163–170 (1998)

Unilateral Laterothoracic Exanthem

Epidemiology

This exanthem is most often seen in children around two years of age, with a range from 6 months to 10 years. There may be a seasonal distribution, with the disorder more common in the spring months, as well as a familial tendency. Girls appear to be more often affected than boys.

Pathogenesis

The most likely explanation for this puzzling clinical pattern is an underlying viral disorder, which would fit with the seasonal pattern and familial clustering. In addition, about 75% of the patients have respiratory signs and symptoms either as a prodrome or accompanying the rash.

Clinical Features

In most instances this clinically distinct exanthem begins in the axilla or groin (Fig. 73). It may spread outside this region, becoming bilateral or disseminated but tends to remain more prominent on one side of the body. The individual lesions are erythematous papules often with a pale periphery. The papules may coalesce and sometimes have a fine scale (Fig. 74). The face, oral mucosa, palms and soles are spared. About two-thirds of the patients have regional lymphadenopathy. The exanthem begins to resolve after about 3 weeks and usually disappears completely by six weeks. In rare cases it may persist for up to four months.

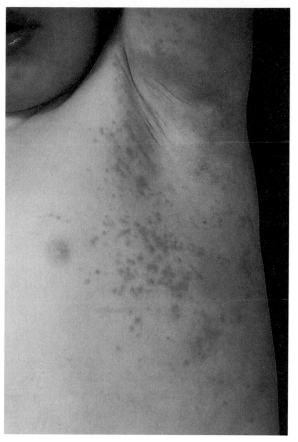

Fig. 73. Unilateral laterothoracic exanthem. Multiple erythematous papules starting in axilla.

Symptoms

The rash may be mildly pruritic. The signs and symptoms associated with the presumed underlying viral infection tend to be mild; high fever is uncommon.

Diagnosis

The diagnosis is clinical. The unilateral nature of the rash usually gives away the answer.

Differential Diagnosis

The differential diagnostic considerations are shown in Table 61.

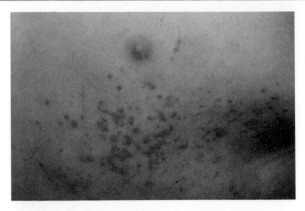

Fig. 74. Unilateral laterothoracic exanthem. Closer view showing confluent papules.

Table 61. Differential diagnosis of unilateral laterothoracic exanthem

Diagnosis	Distinguishing Features
■ **Contact dermatitis**	Erythema, papules and vesicles, accompanied by marked pruritus; generally limited to area of contact with few stray lesions
■ **Pityriasis rosea**	Symmetrically distributed oval erythematous lesions with collarette scale; often larger primary lesion
■ **Scarlet fever**	Velvety pinhead-sized papules begin in the skin folds and spread symmetrically; some are ill with high fever; others have only a mild erythema in area covered by their underpants, as the warmth makes the rash most apparent
■ **Gianotti-Crosti syndrome**	Symmetrical involvement of the extensor surfaces of the extremities, as well as face and buttocks; often associated with viruses (hepatitis B, EBV, CMV)
■ **Tinea corporis**	Patches with peripheral scale and erythema; slowly spreading in centrifugal manner; usually transferred from house pets; KOH and culture positive

Therapy

No therapy is necessary, other than reassuring the parents that the peculiar rash will go away. A bland cream or ointment can be recommended and if pruritus is prominent, a systemic antihistamine given for bedtime use. Topical corticosteroids appear ineffective.

References

Cremer H.J.: Das halbseitenbetonte seitliche Thoraxexanthem. pädiatrische praxis 51:257–262 (1996)

Fölster-Holst R., Christophers E.: Exantheme im Kindesalter. Teil 2: Bakterien- und medikamenteninduzierte Exantheme, Exantheme nach Knochenmarkstransplantation, Exantheme unklarer Ätiopathogenese. Hautarzt 50:601–617 (1999)

Nelson J.S., Stone M.S.: Update on selected viral exanthems. Current Opinion in Pediatrics 12:359–364 (2000)

Mancini A.J.: Exanthems in childhood: An update. Pediatric Annals 27:163–170 (1998)

Strom K., Mempel M., Fölster-Holst R., Abeck D.: Unilaterales laterothorakales Exanthem im Kindesalter – Klinische Besonderheiten und diagnostische Kriterien bei 5 Patienten. Hautarzt 50:39–41 (1999)

■ Erythema Infectiosum

Epidemiology

Erythema infectiosum, also known as fifth disease, is most common seen in children 4 to 10 years of age. Girls are more often affected. There is a seasonal distribution, with most cases seen in the winter and spring.

Pathogenesis

The causative virus is the B19 parvovirus, which is spread by the respiratory droplet route. The illness has an incubation period of 4–15 days. Viral replication occurs in both the peripheral blood and bone marrow where the erythropoetic cells can be damaged. Thus, patients with chronic hemolytic anemia or a hemoglobulinopathy are at risk of aplastic crises, while red cell aplasia has been described in HIV/AIDS patients. In addition, B19 is a dangerous virus during pregnancy, as 1–9% of transplacental infections lead to spontaneous abortions. The greatest risk for hydrops fetalis is between weeks 20–28 of pregnancy.

Clinical Features

The most classical and usually initial sign of erythema infectiosum is a diffuse homogenous erythema of the cheeks (slapped cheek sign) (Fig. 75). A few days later a figurate erythema develops on the distal extremities

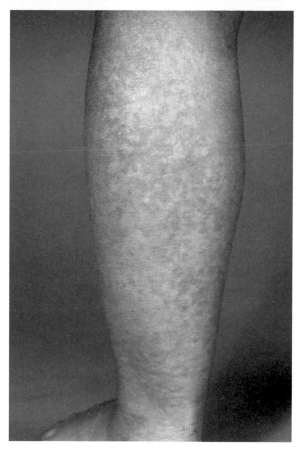

Fig. 76. Erythema infectiosum. Garland or wreath pattern on leg.

and trunk (Fig. 76). The areas of erythema with central clearing produce a wreath or garland pattern. The parents often describe the flaring of the erythema following physical irritation such as sunlight, a warm bath or strenuous physical activity, even as the rash appears to be resolving. This period of waxing and waning lasts for 1 to 3 weeks and is followed by spontaneous resolution. While the child is infectious prior to having the exanthem, the risk of transmission is very low once the skin changes have appeared.

Symptoms

About 15% of the children complain of pruritus. Other signs and symptoms may include malaise, headache, fever, pharyngitis, and

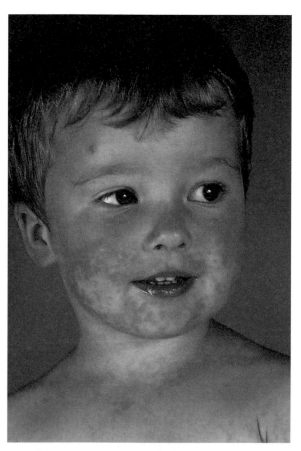

Fig. 75. Erythema infectiosum. Typical erythema of cheeks as well as annular or wreath-like lesions on chin.

gastrointestinal problems. About 10% have arthralgias or arthritis.

Diagnosis

The clinical pattern is so distinct that the diagnosis is easy. It can be confirmed by serology, usually looking for IgM antibodies. High risk individuals (pregnant, HIV/AIDS, hemolytic anemia) should be screened if they have skin lesions suggesting erythema infectiosum or if they have had contact with an infected child. In pregnancy, the amniotic fluid and fetal blood can also be analyzed with PCR looking for viral DNA, as well as IgM antibodies.

■ Differential Diagnosis

The differential diagnostic considerations are shown in Table 62.

Therapy

In most cases, no therapy is needed. If pruritus is severe, systemic antihistamines can be used. Some patients with joint pain may require non-steroidal anti-inflammatory drugs. Once the exanthem appears, the child is no longer infective and can continue to go to kindergarten or school.

Table 62. Differential diagnosis of erythema infectiosum

Diagnosis	Distinguishing Features
■ **Juvenile rheumatoid arthritis**	Transient exanthem, hepatosplenomegaly
■ **Drug-induced exanthem**	History of medication use; more diffuse distribution
■ **German measles (rubella)**	Lymphadenopathy especially occipital and retroauricular; papular exanthem which spreads cranio-caudally

References

Fölster-Holst R., Christophers E.: Exantheme im Kindesalter. Teil 1: Exantheme durch Viren. Hautarzt 50:515–531 (1999)

Nelson J.S., Stone M.S.: Update on selected viral exanthems. Current Opinion in Pediatrics 12:359–364 (2000)

Mancini A.J.: Exanthems in childhood: An update. Pediatric Annals 27:163–170 (1998)

CHAPTER 26 Warts

O. BRANDT

Epidemiology

Warts or verrucae are among the most common infectious skin diseases in children with an incidence of about 10%. The true incidence is probably much higher, as often warts are not clinically identified and in other instances, they heal spontaneously before intervention is sought. Probably every human has at least one wart during the first two decades of life. Warts induce a partial immunity which provides moderate protection against future reinfections.

Pathogenesis

Warts are caused by human papilloma viruses (HPV) and can infect the entire skin surface and mucosa. There are over 100 different types of HPV which lead to a variety of clinical appearances in various locations. Histologically, warts are characterized by a reversible epithelial hyperplasia with characteristic changes of keratinocytes (balloon degeneration producing koilocytes). Common warts (verrucae vulgares) are not surprisingly the most frequently encountered warts; they are usually caused by HPV 1, 2, 4 or less often 7. Plane or flat warts (verrucae planae) are usually associated with HPV 3 or 10.

Warts are usually caused by direct human contact with transfer of HPV but can also be acquired from contaminated objects or surfaces (such as going barefoot in a gymnasium or swimming pool). The papilloma viruses are not strictly species-specific, so that warts caused by feline papilloma virus or canine papilloma virus can be transferred from pets to humans, although this is unusual. Autoinoculation is extremely common, especially with the transfer from the hands to the mouth or perianal region. In addition, whenever warts are arranged linearly, one can guess that they have been transferred by scratching.

The incubation period lasts from several weeks to many months and is influenced by a variety of factors. The two most important are the patient's immune status and condition of their skin. Dermatitis and other skin disorders (for example, tinea pedis, hyperhidrosis, acrocyanosis) allow HPV easier entry to the skin.

Clinical Features

The initial warts in children are most commonly on the fingers or back of the hand. The earliest lesion is a single small sharply defined skin colored papule with a smooth surface. The papule tends to grow rapidly and acquires a rough (or papillomatous) surface reflecting the epithelial hyperplasia and increased keratinization. A characteristic finding in developed warts is tiny dark dots which represent thrombosed capillaries in the papillary dermis (Fig. 77). Patients often refer to these spots as the seeds or roots of the wart. The morphology of a given wart – whether it is papillomatous, filiform (Fig. 78) or mosaic – is to a large extent determined by location and associated me-

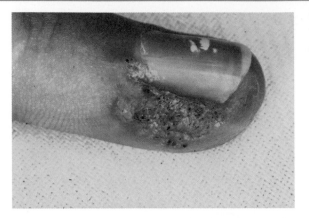

Fig. 77. Common warts. Grouped hyperkeratotic papules with hemorrhagic punctae in typical periungual location.

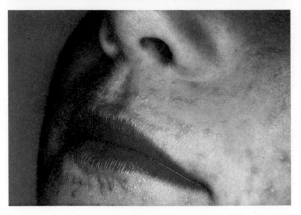

Fig. 79. Plane warts. Numerous red-yellow flat-topped papules. Linear arrangement reflects scratching and Koebner phenomenon.

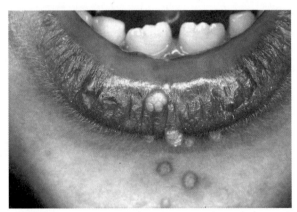

Fig. 78. Common warts. Filiform lesions on lip and chin with complex papillomatous surface.

chanical pressure. Autoinoculation or treatment may lead to numerous small warts arising about the initial larger lesion.

Plantar warts are almost always flat initially because of the obvious mechanical pressure. Multiple plantar warts can fuse together, producing the mosaic pattern. Plantar warts are usually identified by the reactive or protective hyperkeratosis which develops over them, but are marked by numerous dark thrombosed capillaries which sometimes can be better seen as the thickened skin is pared. Their presence helps separate warts from clavi (corns) and calluses.

Plane warts are clinically quite different. They present as small 1–4 mm flat-topped papules, usually skin colored, favoring the face (Fig. 79) but also seen on the distal extremities. Their surface is much smoother than other warts with small indentations rather than distinct papillations.

Symptoms

Common and plane warts are usually asymptomatic or cosmetically disturbing. In contrast, plantar warts frequently are painful and interfere with walking. On rare occasion, other warts may be pruritic.

Diagnosis

The diagnosis is usually made by the patient or parent. Removing the reactive hyperkeratotic skin by gentle paring to reveal the dark spots is an easy way to confirm the diagnosis if confusion exists. Dermatoscopy can also be used to confirm the diagnosis.

Differential Diagnosis

The major differential diagnostic considerations are shown in Table 63.

Table 63. Differential diagnosis of warts

Diagnosis	Distinguishing Features
Common warts	
■ **Verrucous lichen planus**	Hyperkeratotic nodules on erythematous base, on distal extremities, occasionally palms and soles; intensely pruritic; mainly in adults
Plantar warts	
■ **Clavus (corn)**	Small circular hyperkeratotic lesion with a central plug; caused by pressure over a bony exostoses, either over a joint or between the toes; no hemorrhagic punctae
■ **Callus**	Larger, more irregular yellowish hyperkeratotic lesion; results from friction; no hemorrhagic punctae
Plane warts	
■ **Lichen planus**	Smooth dome-shaped violaceous papules; favor wrists; intensely pruritic; lacy white pattern (Wickham streaks) on surface
■ **Lichen nitidus**	Tiny glistening papules usually on penis, neck or inner aspects of arms

Table 64. Treatment of warts

■ **Watchful neglect**	Treatment of choice for warts that are not painful and not a cosmetic problem
■ **Suggestive therapy**	Possible approach without adverse effects in some children
■ **Topical treatment**	
Keratolytic agents	Salicylic acid plasters or solutions Soaking Mechanical trimming or sanding
Anthralin	Anthralin wart paste (see text for Rx) Applied b.i.d. for 10 days Stains, so should be covered, can be very irritating
Glutaraldehyde	10% solution painted on once daily, rinsed after 20 min
Podophyllin	Physician can apply 25% solution 1–2× times weekly or patient can use 0.5% podophyllotoxin solution b.i.d. at home
5-fluorouracil	Solution containing 5FU and salicylic acid available in Europe; apply b.i.d.-t.i.d.
Imiquimod	Apply 5% cream 3× weekly for genital warts; daily or b.i.d. to common warts
Tretinoin	Start with 0.025% cream; may have to work up Apply 1–2× daily to plane warts
■ **Destructive measures**	Cryotherapy Laser destruction Curettage Excision
■ **Systemic therapy**	Cimetidine Dimepranol-inosine

Therapy

Our general therapeutic rule for warts in children is – asymptomatic lesions require no treatment, as spontaneous regression without scarring is the rule. About two-thirds of all children experience such spontaneous resolution of their warts over a two year period. Thus, if the wart is not painful and is not bothering the child, it is appropriate to leave it alone.

If the child is embarrassed by the warts, or if they are painful, then treatment should be undertaken. Even though almost all wart therapy is painful, many children prefer the pain to having the warts. One must be sure that both the child and the parents understand that there is no absolutely effective way of treating warts and that the warts may even worsen during the early stages of treatment. The story is different in immunosup-pressed children, where we tend to treat single or localized lesions early and more aggressively in order to prevent further spreading and more sequelae. The choice of therapy depends on the location, number and type of warts (Table 64).

■ **Suggestive Therapy.** Children, especially those between 5–10 years of age, are generally susceptible to suggestion. If one tells them the wart can be killed with a strong type of light or x-ray and then exposes the lesions to either a Wood light or infrared lamp, therapeutic successes may be observed. To increase the effect, the room can be darkened and special protective glasses provided. Verbal suggestion therapy, encouraging the child to concentrate for 10 minutes every day, perhaps before bedtime, on destroying the wart, is another possibility. Suggestive therapy, which clearly relies on the spontaneous clearing of the wart plus perhaps an enhanced immune response, should not be explained to the child afterwards (but has to be explained to the parents!) or their trust in physicians may be damaged.

■ **Keratolytic-mechanical Therapy.** The easiest and least painful way to physically treat warts is with a keratolytic agent, usually salicylic acid in flexible collodion or in a thick plaster. We prefer the plaster which is cut to be slightly larger than the wart, applied, and covered with tape. On the sole, the pressure of walking dislodges the plaster almost immediately so a sandwich technique is useful. A piece of water-resistant adhesive tape is cut with a central hole just larger than the wart and applied to the skin to leave the wart exposed. Then a generous piece of salicylic acid plaster is applied over the wart and the sandwich is completed with a second intact piece of tape.

After 3–4 days, the plaster is removed and the wart trimmed in the office with a #15 blade or a flexible double edged razor broken in half. If the child is instructed that only dead skin is being removed and that the cutting will stop the minute pain is experienced, tolerance is high. To increase the softening on the sole, the foot can be soaked for 10–20 minutes following removal of the plaster and prior to trimming. At home, the child or parent can trim the wart with a special plane, sanding board or even masonry-type sandpaper.

The liquid wart solutions usually contain salicylic acid and often other irritants in flexible collodion. They must be painted on 1–2 times daily, as they do not adhere as well; the increased time expenditure decreases compliance.

Keratolytic therapy can be combined with many of the other topical measures, such as anthralin paste, glutaraldehyde, imiquimod or even 5-fluorouracil.

■ **Anthralin.** Once the wart has been trimmed (or softened with keratolytics) one can apply an anthralin wart paste, compounded as follows:

Rx_
Anthralin	0.5
Acid salicylic	12.5
Paraffin liquid	2.5
Vaseline ad	50.0

We apply the anthralin wart paste b.i.d. for 10 days. The anthralin cases skin discoloration so the paste should be covered with an adhesive bandage. While some degree of irritation is desired, on occasion the process will burn or cause too much inflammation.

■ **Glutaraldehyde.** Another possibility, especially useful for plantar warts, is to paint the lesions once daily with a 10% glutaraldehyde solution which is left on the skin for 20 minutes and then rinsed off, ideally in combination with soaking in soapy water for 10–15 minutes. Then the hyperkeratotic material is trimmed or sanded. Usually a eight week treatment program is effective in producing a cure. Glutaraldehyde is toxic and not approved for medical use although there are studies on it safety and efficacy. It has to be stored in special containers out of the reach of children.

■ **Podophyllin.** The cytotoxic agent podophyllin has been the mainstay of treating genital warts. While it is less effective on the more keratotic non-genital skin, it may still occasionally be helpful. In the office, one can apply 25% podophyllin in tincture of benzoin, but this concentration should not be provided to the patient. The commercially available product Condylox®, which contains 0.5% podophyllotoxin, is designed for home use but usually elicits little reaction on skin. We occasionally employ it for plane warts.

■ **5-fluorouracil.** Another cytostatic agent, 5-fluorouracil, is combined with 10% salicylic acid in a commercial product (Verrumal®) in Germany. It is applied 2–3 times daily for several weeks. Whether or not it is more effective than salicylic acid alone has never been demonstrated. While the parents fear the side effects of an "dangerous drug", the child only notices that the product is not especially effective.

■ **Imiquimod.** This topical immunomodulator is available as a 5% cream (Aldara®) in Europe and America. While it was also first approved for genital warts, it is also effective for other warts. It has to be combined with a keratolytic regimen and application frequency should be increased to daily or even twice daily instead of 3 times weekly as suggested for genital warts. It is well-tolerated but extremely expensive and not packaged in a standard screw-topped tube, but instead in small foil packets due to limited stability (one day according to the manufacturer, about 3 days from own experience) once opened.

■ **Tretinoin.** Our treatment of choice for plane warts is tretinoin cream or gel. We usually start with the 0.025% cream, but it may be necessary to move up to a stronger cream or gel. The trick is to induce a low grade irritation. The patient applies the tretinoin once daily at night for the first week and then if well-tolerated, increases to a twice daily application. Usually treatment for 4–6 weeks is sufficient.

■ **Cryotherapy.** Another standard approach is cryotherapy. The usual agent is liquid nitrogen which has a temperature of –196 °C. In the case of common warts, keratolytic therapy or trimming should be used first to reduce the amount of dead skin which interferes with the freezing effect. One must freeze deeply enough to induce a subepidermal blister, which as it is shed will include much of the wart.

The freezing does not kill the HPV. Usually a 5–10 second spray perhaps protecting the skin around the wart with a plastic shield or application of a large or modified cotton-tipped applicator dipped in the cryogen is sufficient. An ordinary cotton tip applicator (such as a Q-Tip®) does not take up enough liquid nitrogen to freeze adequately. We prefer to check the wart after 24–48 hours to be sure it has been frozen deeply enough. If not, the process should be repeated. Often patients are seen only every 1–2 weeks, and the treatment never becomes aggressive enough.

Freezing is painful for everyone, but may be too painful for some children, especially on the fingers. It is also not helpful for treating facial lesions (perioral or periorbital) because of the parents' fear of damage. In addition, if one freezes too long or hard, the necrosis may be significant, producing an uncomfortable ulcerated lesion which may become secondarily infected and scar.

We also sometimes use liquid carbon dioxide which has a temperature of only –86 °C for plane warts. Another possibility is just to use a very light freeze with liquid nitrogen, only frosting the warts, not trying to freeze deeply.

■ **Laser Therapy.** A number of lasers can be employed to treat warts. Both the CO_2 and flash lamp pumped dye laser (FPDL) have been shown to be effective. Depending on the location, usually 2–3 treatment cycles are needed at relatively high energy levels. Cure rates between 82–99% have been reported, but long-term follow-up suggests a somewhat less positive picture.

Laser destruction is painful so the warts should be treated with EMLA under occlusion for one hour prior to treatment. If a child has numerous warts or they are in problem areas, general anesthesia may be needed. In addition, appropriate safety measures (masks, exhaust devices) are needed as the laser plume may contain infectious HPV particles.

■ **Surgery.** Minor surgical procedures may also be helpful. Plane warts can be curetted with a sharp curette; in most instances, if the skin is pulled taught and the operator swift, the pain is tolerable. If not, EMLA is once again useful. For larger common warts, local anesthesia plus curettage is also effective. Post-curettage bleeding is common; a variety of hemostatic agents can be employed. We do not treat plantar warts with surgery. The procedure itself is painful, the recurrence rate is very high, and the risk of a painful scar is also great.

■ **Systemic Therapy.** Systemic treatment of warts is used only when local measures are not applicable (too many warts, problem locations) or when topical measures have failed. We usually try either cimetidine or dimepranol-inosine. Cimetidine is an antihistamine which blocks the H2 receptor. Its effectiveness in treating warts is controversial, and there is no satisfactory explanation why it works. We use a dosage of 20–40 mg/kg daily, divided in 3–4 doses, and administered over 4–8 weeks. Side effects are extremely uncommon although some children have been reported with behavioral changes.

Dimepranol-inosine is an immune stimulatory agent, approved for acute viral encephalitis and viral infections in immunosuppressed patients, which we have employed with success in some cases of extremely refractory warts. It is expensive and not available in all parts of the world. The recommended dose is 50 mg/kg daily.

■ **Supportive Measures.** One should remind the parents and patient that warts are infective and that measures should be taken in the home to avoid transmission. Examples include not sharing washcloths, towels, shoes or other items that come in close contact with the warts. Equipment used to trim warts should not be used by other family members until sterilized. Plantar warts should be covered with adhesive tape if a child wants to go barefoot. If the child is participating in contact sports, warts in other areas must also be covered with adhesive tape.

References

Cochrane Database Syst Rev; (2): CD001781 (2001)

Frieden I.J., Penneys N.S.: Papillomavirus, pp. 1281–1286. In: Schachner L.A., Hansen R.C. (eds.) Pediatric Dermatology, 2nd ed. Churchill Livingstone, New York (1995)

Grussendorf-Conen E.I., Jacobs S.: Efficacy of imiquimod 5% cream in the treatment of recalcitrant warts in children. Pediatr Dermatol 19:263–266 (2002)

Siegfried E.: Warts and molluscum on children – an approach to therapy. Dermatologic Therapy 2:51–67 (1997)

Weisshaar E., Gollnick, H.: Potentiating effect of imiquimod in the treatment of verrucae vulgares in immunocomprised patients. Acta Dermato-Venereologica 80:306–307 (2000)

Wimmershoff M.B., Scherer K., Baumler W., Hohenleutner U., Landthaler M.: Treatment of therapy-resistant verruca vulgaris with long-pulsed tunable dye laser. Hautarzt 52:701–704 (2001)

Wiss K.: Warts today – gone tomorrow? Medical and Surgical Dermatology 4:1–4 (1997)

CHAPTER 27 Appendices

Appendix I Choice of Vehicles

Vehicles for topical agents is an issue which rarely concerns physicians other than dermatologist. The vehicle is the cream, ointment or liquid in which an active ingredient is mixed. There is an old saying to the effect that a skilled dermatologist can achieve more by employing the ideal vehicle for a given disease at a certain stage than can an inexperienced physician with the entire spectrum of active ingredients, but no concept of when to use what. It is absolutely crucial to understand the different types of vehicles in which topical medications can be mixed and to employ them with fine touch. In many instances, the drying, lubricating or soothing action of the vehicle plays as great a role as the choice of active ingredients. Conversely, applying exactly the wrong vehicle can countermand even the most appropriately chosen active ingredient. Table 65 lists common vehicles, while Table 66 correlates clinical findings with appropriate and less appropriate vehicles.

In addition to the clinical picture, other factors also influence the choose of a vehicle. They include the skin type of the patient, the location of the lesions and even the season of the year. For example, acne patients with oily skin do better with alcohol-based products, while the uncommon acne patient with dry skin is grateful that water-based products are also available. In general, when the intertriginous areas are treated, oily or greasy products are best avoided. Similarly, any product applied to the scalp must be in a vehicle with can be removed with shampooing. Finally, many patients with atopic dermatitis prefer a greasy vehicle in the winter but a less occlusive product in the summer.

Table 65. Types of vehicles

Vehicle	Description	Common examples
■ **Shake lotion**	Powder dispersed in solution	Zinc oxide shake lotion, calamine lotion
■ **Cream**	Oil in water (o/w) emulsion; oil dispersed in water base	Most disappearing creams; products which patients can "rub in"
■ **Lotion**	Lotions are thin creams	Vaseline Intensive Care Lotion®; many others
■ **Emollient cream**	Water in oil (w/o) emulsion; water dispersed in oily base	Heavier creams, such as Eucerin®
■ **Ointments**	Greasy base; some are hydrophilic (compatible with water)	Hydrophilic= Aquaphor® Hydrophobic=Vaseline®
■ **Pastes**	Powder mixed with cream or ointment; some are absorbent (often called salves in USA)	Zinc oxide paste, many diaper ointments
■ **Gels**	Semisolids that readily become liquids and spread easily; either water or alcohol based	Most products that appear clear or transparent; many acne products

Table 66. Correlation of clinical findings and vehicles

Clinical Finding	Appropriate Vehicles	Inappropriate Vehicles
■ **Erythema**	Shake lotions, wet compresses, creams	Emollient creams, ointments, pastes, powders
■ **Papules and vesicles**	Shake lotions, wet compresses, creams	Emollient creams, ointments, pastes, powders
■ **Excoriated, weeping lesions**	Wet compresses, perhaps combined with an ointment or emollient cream	Ointments, pastes, powders, shake lotions
■ **Intertriginous lesions**	Wet compresses, absorbent pastes	Shake lotions, ointments
■ **Crusted lesions**	Wet compresses combined with an ointment or emollient cream, ointments	Pastes, creams, shake lotions, powders
■ **Chronic lichenified lesions**	Ointments, pastes, w/o creams	o/w creams, solutions, powders, shake lotions
■ **Dry skin**	Creams, ointments, water-based gels	Alcohol-based gels, shake lotions, powders
■ **Oily skin**	Alcohol-based gels, solutions, creams	Ointments, emollient creams

Basic formulations are available both as commercial brand name products and as standard, time-tested formulations which are generic and almost always save money. An advantage in Europe is that many corticosteroid manufacturers provide the corresponding vehicle at a fair price, making it easier to shift the patient between an active ingredient and a vehicle used for long-term care. Patients are attracted to the idea of, for example, using Dermatop® Creme for their atopic dermatitis and then as they improve switching back to Dermatop® Basiscreme.

With compounding, the situation becomes different. There is a still a tendency in Germany to have pharmacists compound dermatologic products. The rationale for this is that active ingredients and vehicles can be optimally combined for the individual patient, and in many instances this can be achieved at less cost than with finished products. It has become clear, though, that this concept is a bit idealized. The products produced by pharmaceutical and cosmetic firms have an optimized vehicle, determined by years of research and testing to be both effective and stable. When other materials,

such as antibiotics, dyes, urea, salicylic acid or a range of agents are added to a finished commercial product, the likelihood is that the pharmacological properties will be altered, sometimes markedly. Thus, one should never add more than one product to a finished product and it should be used in a form which the manufacturer has recommended as compatible. One should not compound in a "free style" fashion but restrict oneself to formulations approved by a national formulary, such as the NRF in Germany or USP in the USA.

References

Abeck D., Cremer H., Pflugshaupt C., Ring J.: Stadienorientierte Auswahl dermatologischer Grundlagen ("Vehikel") bei der örtlichen Therapie des atopischen Ekzems. pädiatrische praxis 52:113–121 (1997)

Pharmazeutisches Laboratorium des „Neues Rezeptur-Formularium"

Standardisierte Rezepturen (NRF/SR) 2001. Govi, Eschborn (2001)

Weston W. L., Lane A. T., Morelli J. G.: Dermatopharmacology and Topical Formulary, pp. 322–331. 3rd edition. Mosby, St. Louis (2002)

Appendix II Prescribing Antibiotics for Children

The principle of prescribing antibiotics for children are not much different from those for adults. One should either have a working diagnosis of an infection, pick an appropriate agent, and be prepared to switch if the clinical course or culture results indicate a microbe is either not present or not responsive to the chosen agent. In children, one must be certain to pick a form that is appropriate for the age of the child and adjust the dosage to the weight (Table 67).

References

Abeck D., Korting H. C., Mempel M.: Pyodermien. Hautarzt 49:243–252 (1998)

Rote Liste Editio Cantor, Aulendorff (2001)

Epstein M. E., Amodio-Groton M., Sadick N. S.: Antimicrobial agents for the dermatologist. I. -lactam antibiotics and related compounds. Journal of the American Academy of Dermatology 37: 149–165 (1997)

Epstein M. E., Amodio-Groton M., Sadick N. S.: Antimicrobial agents for the dermatologist. II. Macrolides, fluoroquinolones, rifamycins, tetracyclines, trimethoprim-sulfamethoxazole, and clindamycin. Journal of the American Academy of Dermatology 37:365–381 (1997)

Gloor M., Ringelmann R.: Antibiotika in der Dermatologie. Zeitschrift für Haut- und Geschlechtskrankheiten 71:672–677 (1996)

Simon C., Stille W.: Antibiotika-Therapie in Klinik und Praxis, 10. Auflage. Schattauer, Stuttgart New York (2000)

Table 67. Important antibiotics for pediatric dermatology

Antibiotic	Form	Size	Dosage
Penicillins			
■ Penicillin V (phenoxymethyl PCN)	Liquid	60,000 IU/mL	Newborn: 100,000 IU 2–3×daily Infant: 150,000 IU t.i.d. 1–6 years: 300,000 IU t.i.d. >6 years: 500,000 IU t.i.d.
	Tablet	400,000–1,500,000 IU	
■ Benzathine PCN V	Liquid	150,000 IU/mL	Infant: 187,500 IU b.i.d. 1–6 years: 375,000 IU t.i.d. >6 years: 750,000 IU t.i.d.
	Tablet	1,500,000 IU	
■ Amoxicillin	Liquid	50 mg/mL	<5 kg: 125–250 mg q.i.d. 5–10 kg: 250–500 mg q.i.d. 10–15 kg: 375–750 mg q.i.d. 15–20 kg: 500–1000 mg q.i.d. >6 years: 1–2 g t.i.d.
	Tablet	250–500–1000 mg	
Penicillinase-resistant penicillin			
■ Flucloxacillin	Liquid	50 mg/mL	0–6 years 40–50 mg/kg daily 6–10 years: 750 mg–1.5 g daily 10–14 years: 1.5–2.0 g daily >14 years: 3.0 g daily *in each case, in 3 divided doses*
	Capsule	250, 500 mg	
Cephalosporins			
■ Cephalexin	Liquid	50 mg/mL	0–14 years: 25–100 mg/kg daily >14 years: 1.5–3.0 g daily *in each case, in 3 divided doses*
	Tablet	500 mg–1.0 g	
■ Cefuroximaxetil	Liquid	25 mg/mL	3 mo.–5 years: 20 mg/kg daily *in two divided doses* 5–12 years: 250 mg b.i.d. >12 years: 500 mg b.i.d.
	Tablet	125, 250, 500 mg	
Macrolides			
■ Erythromycin	Liquid	40–80 mg/mL	30–50 mg/kg daily *in 2–4 divided doses*
	Tablet or capsule	250–500–1000 mg	
■ Roxithromycin	Tablet	50 mg	7–13 kg: 25 mg b.i.d. 14–26 kg: 50 mg b.i.d. 27–40 kg: 100 mg b.i.d. >40 kg: 150 mg b.i.d. or 300 mg daily *always before meals*
	Tablets	150, 300 mg	

Appendices II
– Antibiotics –

Table 67 (continued)

Antibiotic	Form	Size	Dosage
■ Clarithromycin	Liquid	25 mg/mL 50 mg/mL	6 mo.–2 years: 62.5 mg b.i.d. 2–4 years: 125 mg b.i.d. 4–8 years: 187.5 mg b.i.d. 8–12 years: 250 mg b.i.d. >12 years: 500 mg b.i.d.
	Tablet	250, 500 mg	
Lincosamides			
■ Clindamycin	Liquid	15 mg/mL	10–20 mg/kg daily *in 3–4 divided doses*
	Capsule	75, 150, 300 mg	>14 years: 1.2–2.7 g *in 3–4 divided doses*

Appendix III Prescribing Antihistamines for Children

Antihistamines are widely used in treating childhood skin diseases. There are a number of different agents available; those which we most commonly employ are shown in Table 68.

The main indications for antihistamines are urticaria and pruritus, as well as for other aspects of the atopic disease complex, such as allergic rhinitis and conjunctivitis. They are considerably more effective for the itching associated with urticaria than for other types of pruritus. For example, in atopic dermatitis which is highly pruritic, some feel that the main effect of antihistamines is sedation, not blocking of histamine. In each instance, the sedating effect of the substance must be considered. In addition, there are age limits below which the various agents are not recommended. In our practice, we favor the non-sedating agents such as loratadine and cetirizine, especially during the day in school age children. We no longer employ terfenadine because of drug safcty issues. The older sedating antihistamines can be used in the evenings or when alertness is not as crucial. Two new non-sedating agents, descarboxyloratadine and levocetirizine hydrochloride, have also proved useful for children over 2 years of age.

While antihistamines are very safe medications, they have a complex range of drug interactions. Thus, it is always crucial to find out if a child is taking any other drugs before prescribing an antihistamine. The best known side effect is the triggering of ventricular extrasystoles when antihistamines and other drugs metabolized by isoenzyme 3A4 of cytochrome P450 are combined. Included in this group are terfenadine, hydroxyzine, macrolide antibiotics (especially erythromycin, seldom clarithromycin, not azithromycin) and imidazoles (fluconazole, itraconazole). In addition, some antihistamines have a paradoxical effect in children, making them hyperactive rather than somnolent.

References

Abeck D., Werfel S., Brockow K., Ring J.: Die Behandlung des atopischen Ekzems im Kindesalter. Hautarzt 48:379–383 (1998)

Diepgen T.L.: Long-term treatment with cetirizine of infants with atopic dermatitis: a multi-country, double-blind, randomized, placebo-controlled trial (the ETAC trade mark trial) over 18 months. Pediatr Allergy Immunol 13:278–286 (2002)

Reider N., Zloczower M., Fritsch P., Kofler H.: Antihistaminika, Teil ;I. Hautarzt 49:674–681 (1998)

Reider N., Zloczower M., Fritsch P., Kofler H.: Antihistaminika, Teil II. Hautarzt 49:734–742 (1998)

Simons F.E.: H1-antihistamines in children. Clin Allergy Immunol 17:437–464 (2002)

Appendices III
– Antihistamines –

Table 68. Important antihistamines for pediatric dermatology

Agent	Age	Form	Size	Dosage
Sedating				
■ Clemastine hydrogen fumarate	>1 yr	Liquid	0.67 mg/10 mL	1–3 yr: 1–2 teasp. b.i.d. 4–6 yr: 2 teasp. b.i.d. 7–12 yr: 1 tablsp. b.i.d. >12 yr: 1½; tablsp. b.i.d.
		Tablet	1.34 mg	4–6 yr: ½; tab. b.i.d. 7–12 yr. ½–1 tab. b.i.d. >12 yr: 1 tab. b.i.d.
■ Dimethindene maleate	all	Liquid	0.122 mg/mL	0–8 yr: 1 teasp. t.i.d. >8 yr: 1½; teasp. t.i.d.
		Drops	1 mg/mL (20 drops)	0–8 yr: 10-15 drops t.i.d. >8 yr: 20 drops t.i.d.
		Dragee	1 mg	>3 yr: 1 dragee t.i.d.
■ Doxylamine succinate	>2 yr	Syrup	6.25 mg/5 mL	>2 yr: 1–2 tsp. 1–3×daily
■ Hydroxyzine	6 yr	Liquid	10 mg/5 mL	6–10 yr: 25–50 mg daily >10 yr: 37.5–75 mg daily
		Tablet	25 mg	6–10 yr: 1–2 tabs. daily >10 yr: 1½–3 tabs. daily
Non-sedating				
■ Cetirizine	>1 yr	Liquid	1 mg/mL	1–12 yr, <30 kg: 1 teasp. h.s. >12 yr or >30 kg: 2 teasp. h.s.
		Drops	10 mg/mL (20 drops)	1–12 yr, <30 kg: 10 drops. h.s. >12 yr or >30 kg: 20 drops h.s.
		Tablet	10 mg	2–12 yr, <30 kg: ½ tab. h.s. >12 yr or >30 kg: 1 tab. h.s.
■ Loratadine	2 yr	Syrup	5 mg/5 mL	2–12 yr, <30 kg: 1 teasp. daily >12 yr or >30 kg: 2 teasp. daily
		Dissolving tablet	10 mg	2–12 yr, <30 kg: ½ tab. daily >12 yr or >30 kg: 1 tab. daily
		Tablet	10 mg	2–12 yr, <30 kg: ½ tab. daily >12 yr or >30 kg: 1 tab. daily
■ Descarboxy loratadine	2 yr	Tablet		1 tab. daily
■ Levocetirizine hydrochloride	2 yr	Tablet		1 tab. daily

Appendix IV Prescribing Topical Corticosteroids for Children

Topical corticosteroids are the mainstay of treating of most inflammatory dermatoses. There are a wide variety of agents available which are ranked in Germany in four different strength groups (classes I–IV with IV being the strongest; Table 69). This ranking is in contrast to that employed in the USA which follows the criteria of Cornell and Stoughton, (classes 1–7 with 1 being most potent).

In addition to the potency of the agent, one must consider the vehicle. The right corticosteroid in the wrong vehicle will do little to help the patient. In addition, a sufficient amount should be prescribed to complete the recommended treatment plan. For example, telling a mother to treat her child's widespread atopic dermatitis each evening with a mid-potency corticosteroid and providing only a 15 gram tube is not much better than doing nothing.

In pediatric patients, the high-potency agents are only occasionally used. The potential cutaneous side effects include erythema, telangiectases, atrophy, hypertrichosis and striae. Corticosteroids are better absorbed in children and also have a greater potential for systemic action because of the different ratio of skin surface to body weight. Maximum absorption occurs in the genital area and on the face where extra care must be observed.

For many years, the idea of identifying topical corticosteroids where the risk of side effects did not correlate with the efficacy was a dream. In other words, as one developed a stronger agent, it almost invariably had more side effects. In the past decade, a number of agents have been developed which have much more favorable risk:benefit ratios. These agents are known as fourth generation corticosteroids. They are all chemical compounds which can be viewed as prodrugs activated by splitting the 21-ester bond. The skin is able to accomplish this conversion easily with its available esterases. Agents in this group include hydrocortisone aceponate, hydrocortisone buteprate, hydrocortisone butyrate, methylprednisolone aceponate and prednicarbate. These substances are also designated "soft drugs", because they are metabolized in the skin in a first pass effect to forms which are not active systemically. Thus, when they are used appropriately, no side effects, either cutaneous or systemic, are observed. Not surprisingly, they have become well-established in pediatric dermatology.

In almost all instances, a single daily application of corticosteroids is sufficient. A reservoir of corticosteroids build up in the stratum corneum from which they are released. The treated area should be handled again after a few hours with a non-medicated basic cream or ointment.

Literatur

Korting H.C.: Dermatotherapie. Springer, Berlin (1995)

Niedner R. (Hrsg.): Kortikoide in der Dermatologie. UNI-MED, Bremen (1998)

Appendices IV
– Topical Corticosteroids –

Table 69. German classification of topical corticosteroids

Active Ingredient	Conc. %	Brand Names
Class I (*weakest*)		
Hydrocortisone	0.5–1.0	Many
Hydrocortisone-21-acetate	0.5–2.5	Many
Prednisolone	0.4	Linola-H N, Linola-H Fett N
Fluocortinbutylester	0.75	Vaspit
Class II		
Methylprednisolone aceponate	0.1	Advantan
Hydrocortisone aceponate	0.1	Retef
Triamcinolone acetonide	0.025–0.1	Volon, many others
Fluprednidene-21-acetate	0.1	Decoderm
Hydrocortisone butyrate	0.1	Alfason
Hydrocortisone buteprate	0.1	Pandel
Betamethasone-17-valerate	0.05	Betnesol-V mite
Prednicarbate	0.25	Dermatop
Desoximetasone	0.05	Topisolon mite
Class III		
Betamethasone-17-valerate	0.1	Betnesol-V
Betamethasone-17,21-dipropionate	0.05	Diprosone
Diflucortolone-21-valerate	0.1	Nerisona
Class IV (*strongest*)		
Diflucortolone-21-valerate	0.3	Nerisona forte
Clobetasol-17-propionate	0.05	Dermoxin

Subject Index

Printing and Binding: Stürtz AG, Würzburg